Optavia Diet Cookbook

2021

A Complete Simple Guide on How to Use Optavia Diet to Lose Weight Faster and in an Easy Way | The New Weight Loss Program 5 & 1.

Patricia Ramos

TABLE OF CONTENTS

INTRODUCTION 4

CHAPTER I: WHAT IS THE OPTAVIA DIET? 7

CHAPTER II: A DETAILED LOOK AT THE OPTAVIA DIET 24

CHAPTER III: BENEFITS OF OPTAVIA DIET 30

CHAPTER IV: THE OPTAVIA DIET GUIDE 38

CHAPTER V: MORE INFO ABOUT OPTAVIA DIET 50

CHAPTER VI: RECIPES FOR BREAKFAST 57

CHAPTER VIII: SNACK FOOD 106

CHAPTER IX: LEAN AND GREEN RECIPES 138

CHAPTER X: MEAT AND FISH DISHES 183

CONCLUSION 224

Introduction

The Optavia diet concept was introduced by the team behind Medifast, a famous meal replacement company. Following the Optavia program requires you to feed on low calorie and reduced carb foods. You will need a combination of packaged foods and homemade meals to lose weight effectively. If you don't enjoy cooking or are a busy type and don't have enough time to cook your meals, the Optavia diet will be great for you as it doesn't require you to do prolonged cooking.

It is important to note that while Medifast does not require one-on-one coaching, the Optavia diet requires.

Optavia diet enhances weight loss through branded products known as fueling, while the homemade entrées are referred to as the Lean and Green meals. The fuelings are made up of over 60 items, specifically low carbs but are high in probiotic cultures and Protein. The fuelings ultimately contain friendly bacteria that can help to boost gut health. They include; cookies, bars, puddings, shakes, soups, cereals, and pasta.

Looking at the listed foods, you might think they are quite high in carbs; that is understandable, but the fuelings are composed in such a way that they are lower in sugar and carbs than the traditional versions of similar foods. The company does this by using small portion sizes and sugar substitutes. Many of the fuelings are packed with soy protein isolate and whey protein powder in furtherance. Those interested in the Optavia diet plan but are not interested or got no chance to cook are provided with pre-made low-carb meals. These meals are referred to as Flavors of Home, and they can sufficiently replacing the Lean and Green Meals.

The company explicitly states that by working with its team of coaches and following the Optavia diet as required, you will achieve a "lifelong transformation, one healthy habit at a time."

Therefore, to record success with this diet plan, you have to stick to the fuelings supplemented by veggie, meat, and healthy fat entrée daily; you will be full and nourished. Although you will be consuming low calories, you will not be losing a lot of muscle since you will be feeding on lots of fiber, protein, and other vital nutrients. Your calories as an adult will not exceed 800-1,000. You can lose 12 pounds in 12 weeks if you follow the optimal weight 5&1 plan option.

Since you will curb your carb intake while on this diet plan, you will naturally shed fat because the carb is the primary source of energy; therefore if it is not readily available, the body finds a fat alternative, which implies that the body will have to break down your fats for energy and keep burning fat.

Summary: The Optavia diet is an idea of Medifast, and it comprises of pre-purchased portioned snacks and meals, low carb Lean and Green (homemade) meals, and continuous coaching that is based on facilitating fat and weight loss.

Chapter I: What is the Optavia Diet?

The famous meal replacement company. Following the Optavia program requires you to feed on low calorie and reduced carb foods. You will need the Optavia diet concept was introduced by the team behind Medifast, a combination of packaged foods and homemade meals, to lose weight effectively. If you don't enjoy cooking or are a busy type and don't have enough time to cook your meals, the Optavia diet will be great for you as it doesn't require you to do prolonged cooking.

It is important to note that while Medifast does not require one-on-one coaching, the Optavia diet requires.

Optavia diet enhances weight loss through branded products known as fueling, while the homemade entrées are referred to as the Lean and Green meals. The fuelings are made up of over 60 items that are specifically low carbs but are high in probiotic cultures and protein. The fuelings ultimately contain friendly bacteria that can help to boost gut health. They include; cookies, bars, puddings, shakes, soups, cereals, and pasta.

Looking at the listed foods, you might think they are quite high in carbs, which is understandable, but the fuelings are composed so that they are lower in sugar and carbs than the traditional versions of similar foods. The company does this by using small portion sizes and sugar substitutes. Many of the fuelings are packed with soy protein isolate and whey protein powder in furtherance. Those interested in the Optavia diet plan but are not interested or got no chance to cook are provided with pre-made low-carb meals. These meals are referred to as Flavors of Home, and they can sufficiently replace the Lean and Green Meals.

The company explicitly states that by working with its team of coaches and following the Optavia diet as required, you will achieve a "lifelong transformation, one healthy habit at a time."

Therefore, to record success with this diet plan, you have to stick to the fuelings supplemented by veggie, meat, and healthy fat entrée daily—you will be full and nourished. Although you will be consuming low calories, you will not be losing a lot of muscle since you will be feeding on lots of fiber, protein, and other vital nutrients. Your calories as an adult will not exceed 800-1,000. You can lose 12 pounds in 12 weeks if you follow the optimal weight 5&1 plan option.

Since you will curb your carb intake while on this diet plan, you will naturally shed fat because the carb is the primary source of energy; therefore if it is not readily available, the body finds a fat alternative, which implies that the body will have to break down your fats for energy and keep burning fat.

The Optavia diet is an idea of Medifast. It comprises pre-purchased portioned snacks and meals, low carb Lean and Green (homemade) meals, and continuous coaching based on facilitating fat and weight loss.

Optavia is a weight reduction or maintenance strategy that prescribes consuming a combination of imported, refined meals—called "fueling"—and "healthy and fresh" prepared meals. There are no sugars and no calories to register. Followers often apply water to dried food or unpack a bar as parts of six-or-so small meals a day. Optavia also provides instructor advice to help you understand the copyrighted "Habits of Fitness."

However, the package advises that you perform approximately 30 minutes of moderately intense workout every day.

The Optavia diet is a high-protein diet, including protein contributing 10–35 percent of the calories a day. But the dried, powdered kind may have some less-than-pleasant results.

"Protein extract with additives will render people feel bloated or have some certain unpleasant GI side effects making you best off in a smoothie with sugar-free Greek protein yogurt," says London.

Moreover, the FDA does not control the protection and effectiveness of

dietary supplements such as shakes and powders the same way it does with food. "Powders and protein 'blends' may have unhealthy additives, or could interfere with a drug you might be taking," says London, "making it especially critical to be sure that your doctor understands you are following the diet."

To encourage weight reduction, Optavia depends on intensively limiting calories. Both of the "fuelings" are about 100–110 calories each, which ensures you will consume only 1,000 calories a day on this diet.

London believes that there is a healthier solution to sustainable weight loss: "Consuming meals and snacks that contain lots of vegetables, 100% whole grains, almonds, beans, legumes, and pulses, low-fat dairy goods, meat, fish, and lean beef with few indulgences is the perfect way to lose weight for the long haul sustainably."

Under the name OPTAVIA, the group behind Medifast has launched a new product line with the same macronutrient composition as the previous Medifast goods. The organization claims that you'll experience "lifelong improvement, one good change at a time" by engaging with its coaching and adopting a lifestyle with Optavia items.

More importantly, you can remain complete and nourished if you adhere to the brand's goods named "Fuelings" and replace them with a meat, vegetable, and balanced fat entrée per day. You would still not lose tons of muscle since you can consume plenty of calcium, fiber, and essential nutrients while eating relatively little calories—usually between 800 and 1,000 for adults. Customers on the Optimum Weight 5&1 Package drop an average of around 12 pounds every 12 weeks.

There is even some carb curbing in behind the scenes. Since carbs are the primary sources of energy, limiting them takes the body to the best substitute fuel available: fat. OPTAVIA is advised to reduce the carbohydrates just enough to start losing fat—you'll consume 80 to 100 grams a day.

Medifast Inc. is Optavia's parent organization. It still manages and maintains the Medifast service that you can recall from the 80s and 90s, which saw physicians recommending meals for their patients. Optavia provides common foods with an equivalent macronutrient profile, so customers should sign up directly for the package themselves.

Possible Benefits of Optavia Diet

The Optavia diet has many benefits that can be achieved when practiced according to its "stern" guidelines. Some of the benefits are:

Is Easy to Follow

Taking the diet is very easy as it relies mainly on prepackaged fuelings, and out of all of the 6 meals, you will need to take per day, while on the 5&1 plan, you will only need to cook only 1 of the meals.

For any plan you decide to take, you will be provided with a sample meal plan and meal logs to help you keep to the diet.

You can only cook a maximum of 1-3 Lean and green meals daily based on the type of plan you are taking, and these meals are straightforward to make. You will be given a list of food options and specific recipes you can always choose from.

Those who are engaged and too busy to cook but wish to take on the Optavia diet plan can still practice it with ease as there is an option to buy packaged meals, which are referred to as Flavors of Home; this can replace the Lean and Green meals.

It Helps to Improve Blood Pressure

The programs can also help improve patients' blood pressure by losing weight and low sodium intake. Optavia meals are well made. They provide below 2,300mg of sodium per day, the recommended consumption level of sodium per day by the United States Department of Agriculture (USDA).

It Helps to Lose Weight

The diet contributes/helps people who actively desire to lose weight and excess fat. It does this by reducing the number of calories and carbs taken in through its well-controlled portion meals and snacks. Studies have shown that a reduction in overall calorie intake can result in a more significant weight loss; this is when full or partial meal replacement habits accompany it.

Coaches Offer Their Support

Health coaches involved in Optavia dieting are often available for consultation throughout losing weight or maintaining one's weight. And research has shown that having access to a lifestyle coach can aid long-term weight maintenance as time goes on.

Ability to Improve Blood Pressure

The Optavia diet program can improve participants' blood pressure since low sodium consumption and weight loss.

Most Optavia meals will not give you more than 2,300mg of sodium daily.

Several health organizations such as the American Heart Association, Institute of Medicine, and the United States Department of Agriculture (USDA) have already given recommendations on consuming less than 2,300mg of sodium daily since higher sodium consumption can increase the risk of developing heart disease and high blood pressure in salt-sensitive people.

Ongoing Support

Once you subscribe to the Optavia program, you will have access to the coach assigned to you throughout the programs' cause. This is valid for whichever plan you put up for, either for weight maintenance or loss. The numerous coaching sessions associated with the program have significantly enhanced weight loss among the program participants.

Low sodium intake that lowers the risk of blood pressure and heart disease, lifestyle coach support that has been effective in achieving significant weight loss and maintenance, the flexibility of the meal plans which makes it easy to follow, ability to lose excess weight and fats in few and much more are some of the benefits you can get by subscribing to the Optavia diet program.

Possible Downsides of the Optavia Diet

Although the Optavia diet is an effective weight-loss tool, it has some potential disadvantages. Some of its downsides are:

Meager Calorie Consumption

The Optavia diet only room for only 800-1,200 calories consumed daily while on the 5&1 plan, which is very low for an adult consuming more than 2,000 calories before then.

Even though the low-calorie intake can significantly result in weight loss, it can also lead to muscle loss.

Studies have shown that low-calorie diets can lead to frequent hunger and cravings, making adhering to the diet plan more difficult.

It Can Be Challenging to Stick With

The 5&1 plan of the Optavia diet program includes 5 prepackaged fuelings and 1 Lean and Green meal (low carb) only. This shows that the program has restricted food options and low-calorie count; hence, it can be difficult to stick by it. Since the food options are restricted and not what you are used to, you can get tired along the line while on the program, and as such, you can easily develop cravings for other foods and cheat on the diet.

Even though the maintenance plan is not as restrictive as the other 2 control plans, it also depends mainly on fuelings.

The Optavia Diet Program Can Be Expensive

The Optavia diet can be costly regardless of which of the plan you chose.

An average of 3 weeks' worth of Optavia fuelings can be in the region of 120 servings, while on the 5&1 plan can cost between $350-$450. However, this cost will also include the coaching for that period, but it does not cover the cost of groceries for the recommended Lean and Green meals.

Why and How Is Optavia Diet Better Than Keto and Other Diets?

While the keto diet often significantly limits carb consumption, much of the diet is made up of fats and protein. The Keto diet was initially meant for people suffering from neuro psychosis.

Whereas the rest of the food in the Optavia diet is prepackaged, highly refined, filled with chemical agents and sweeteners. Yeah, much of the food you consume is unhealthy, refined, and costly too.

If you choose to shed weight more efficiently and comfortably, Optavia will be your nutritional go-to. But you'll bear the chance of severe dietary malnutrition, muscle weakness, and mental health disorders at the same time. This lifestyle could prove ineffective, toxic, and pretty costly for you in the long run. You can lose the lost weight since it is challenging to sustain long-term value with this diet and not researched.

Is Optavia a Diet containing Ketogenic? No, this diet isn't like the ketogenic diet, an incredibly low-carbohydrate plan. You are consuming many fats on a keto diet, a small amount of protein, and relatively little carbohydrates. The meal plan converts into consuming fruit next to no, hardly any grains like rice and bread, and plenty of high-fat foods like avocado, beef, and olive oil.

Optavia 's software might be a good match for you if you want a simple and easy-to-follow diet plan that helps you lose weight easily and includes comprehensive social support.

The Convenience Offered by Packaged Products

The mixes, soups, and other such meal replacement items from Optavia are shipped straight to your door—a degree of comfort not provided by many other diets.

While you'll need to search for your own recipes for "healthy and green" foods, Optavia's "fuelings" home delivery service saves time and resources.

When the goods arrive, they make great grab-and-go foods and are simple to cook.

Achieves Instant Weight Loss

Many healthy people need around 1500 to 3000 calorie intake per day to keep their weight going. Restricting the amount to as little as 800 effectively means that most people lose weight.

Optavia's 5 & 1 package is tailored for accelerated weight reduction, making it a great choice to quickly lose pounds on those with a legitimate condition.

Ends Guesswork

Some people find the worst aspect of dieting to be the personal work needed to sort out what to consume every day—or even at a meal.

Optavia soothes the burden of meal preparation and "decision exhaustion" by providing consumers clear-cut accepted meals with "fuelings" and "healthy and green" menu recommendations.

Simply because of how little calories its fuelings and "healthy and fresh" meals contain, the Optavia Diet may be more efficient for fast weight loss than other strategies.

The USA 2019 The Optavia Diet was rated 31st in Best Diets Overall by News and World Report Best Diets, earning a combined score of 2.7/5.

Optavia needs fewer "technical gymnastics" than competitions, including Weight Watchers (for which you need to develop a target system) or keto (for which you need to observe and measure macronutrients carefully).

The coaching aspect of Optavia is similar to that of Jenny Craig and Weight Watchers, urging people to opt-in for peer group meetups.

Compared to the variety of new, organic foods you can consume on more self-guided diets like Atkins, the heavily refined quality of most things you'll consume on the Optavia diet may be a drawback.

Although the 5 & 1 schedule for Optavia is meant for weight loss, the intake of 800 to 1000 calories a day is a drastic reduction in the USDA's advice.

One field where Optavia deviates from USDA guidelines is in terms of macronutrients—carbohydrates explicitly.

The designs for Optavia potentially have 80 to 100 grams of carbohydrates a day. In other terms, roughly 40 percent of the diet's total calories come from sugars, whereas the USDA Dietary Recommendations prescribe a diet of 45 to 65 percent carbohydrates.

The USDA further stresses that a balanced eating schedule involves grains and dairy items not included in the 5 & 1 package for Optavia.

Chapter II: A detailed look at the Optavia diet

They should take daily. To make this possible, dieters are motivated to choose healthier food items and meal replacements. But unlike otherheOptaviaDietencouragespeopletolimitthenumber ofcaloriesthat types of commercial diet regimens, the Optavia Diet comes in three different variations that one can choose according to their needs.

Various Optavia Diet Plans

5&1 Optavia diet plan: This is the most common version of the Optavia Diet. This one includes consuming five pre-packed meals from them and one home-made balanced dinner.

4&2&1 Optavia diet plan: This diet plan is designed for people who want to have flexibility while following this regimen. Under this program, dieters are encouraged to eat more calories and have more flexible food choices. It means that they can finish four pre-packed Optimal Health Fuelings food, three home-cooked meals from the Lean and Green, and one snack daily.

5&2&2 Optavia diet plan: This diet plan is perfect for individuals who prefer to have a flexible one to achieve a healthy weight. It is recommended for a wide variety of people. Under this diet regimen, dieters must eat five fuelling, two lean and green meals, and two healthy snacks.

3&3 Optavia diet plan: This diet plan is created for people who have moderate weight problems and merely want to maintain a healthy body. Under this diet plan, dieters are encouraged to consume three prepackaged Optimal Health Fuelings and three home-cooked meals.

Optavia for nursing mothers: This diet regimen is designed for nursing mothers with babies of at least two months old. Aside from supporting breastfeeding mothers, it also encourages gradual weight loss.

Optavia for diabetes: This Optavia Diet plan is designed for people who have type 1 and type 2 diabetes. The meal plans are developed so that dieters consume more green and lean meals, depending on their needs and condition.

Optavia for gout: This diet regimen incorporates a balance of low in purines and moderate in protein.

Optavia for seniors (65 years and older): this is designed for seniors. The Optavia Diet plan has some variations following the components of fuelings, depending on the senior dieters' needs and activities.

Optavia for teen boys and for teen girls (13–18 years old): Designed for active teens, the Optavia for Teens Boys and Optavia for Teens Girls provide the right nutrition to growing teens.

Regardless of which type of Optavia Diet plan you choose, you must talk with someone to coach you. He will assist you in determining which method is right for you based on your individual goals. It is to ensure that you get the most out of the program you have chosen.

How to Start This Diet

The Optavia Diet is comprised of different phases. A certified coach will educate you on the steps you need to undertake to follow this regimen. Considering those people who are new to this diet, below are some of the matters that you need to know when starting with this diet regimen.

How to Manage This Diet

During this phase, people are encouraged to consume 800 to 1,000 calories to help you shed off at least 12 pounds within the next 12 weeks. For instance, if you are following the 5&1 Optavia Diet Plan, you need to eat one meal every 2 or 3 hours and include a 30-minute moderate workout on most days of your week. You need to consume not more than 100 grams of carbs daily during this phase.

Further, consuming the Lean and Green meals are highly encouraged. It involves eating 5 to 7 ounces of cooked lean proteins, three servings of non-starchy vegetables, and two healthy fats. This phase also encourages the dieter to include one optional snack per day, such as ½-cup sugar-free gelatin, three celery sticks, and 12 ounces nuts. Aside from these things, below are other things that you need to remember when following this phase:

Make sure that the portion size recommendations are for cooked weight and not the raw one of your ingredients.

Opt for meals that are baked, grilled, broiled, or poached. Avoid frying foods, as this will increase your calorie intake.

You need to consume fish that are rich in Omega-3 fatty acids, at least two servings. These include fishes like tuna, salmon, trout, mackerel, herring, and other cold-water fishes.

Choose meatless alternatives like tofu and tempeh.

Follow the program even when you are dining out. Keep in mind that drinking alcohol is discouraged when following this plan.

How to Maintain the Desired Results

When you reach your weight goals, the next phase is the transition stage. It is a 6-week stage that involves increasing your calorie intake to 1,550 per day. You can also add more varieties into your meal, such as whole grains, low-fat dairy, and fruits.

After six weeks, you can now move into the 3&3 Optavia Diet plan, so you must eat three Lean and Green meals and 3 Fueling foods.

Chapter III: Benefits of Optavia diet

The Optavia diet has additional focal points that may uphold weight decrease and prosperity when all is said in done.

Steps to follow:

As the diet generally relies upon prepackaged Fuelings, you're only subject to setting one up supper for consistently on the 5&1 Plan.

Moreover, every plan goes with dinner logs, and test supper expects to make it less complex to follow.

While you're asked to cook 1–3 Lean and Green suppers consistently, dependent upon the course of action, they're anything but difficult to make — as the program joins express plans and a once-over of food choices.

Also, the people who aren't enthusiastic about getting ready can buy packaged dinners called Flavors of Home to displace Lean and Green suppers.

May Improve Blood Circulatory

Optavia ventures may help improve circulatory strain through weight decrease and confined sodium utilization.

While the Optavia diet hasn't been investigated expressly, a 40-week move in 90 people with excess weight or heaviness on a similar Medifast program revealed a tremendous abatement in circulatory strain.

Additionally, all Optavia feast plans are expected to give under 2,300 mg of sodium for consistently — regardless of the way that it's reliant upon you to pick low sodium decisions for Lean and Green dinners.

Different prosperity affiliations, including the Institute of Medicine, American Heart Association, and the United States

Department of Agriculture (USDA), recommend using under 2,300 mg of sodium per day.

That is because higher sodium affirmation is associated with an extended threat of hypertension and coronary disease in salt-delicate individuals.

Offers Advancing Help

Optavia's prosperity guides are available all through the weight decrease and upkeep programs.

As noted more than, one examination found an essential association between the number of training gatherings on the Optavia 5&1 Plan and improved weight decrease.

In addition, research suggests that having a lifestyle coach or promoter may help long stretch weight uphold.

Expected Drawbacks of Optavia Diet

While the Optavia diet may be an effective weight decrease procedure for a couple, it has a couple of anticipated downsides.

Low in Calories

With just 800–1,2000 calories for consistently, the Optavia 5&1 program is low in calories, especially for individuals who are familiar with eating at any rate 2,000 consistently.

While this quick lessening in calories may achieve all in all weight decrease, research has shown that it can incite enormous muscle incident.

Additionally, low-calorie diets may decrease the number of calories your body devours by as much as 23%.

May Be Contrary to Other Eating Plans

The Optavia diet consolidates explicit undertakings for veggie darlings, people with diabetes, and breastfeeding women. In addition, around 66% of its things are certified sans gluten. Regardless, options are obliged for those on express diets.

For example, Optavia Fuelings are not proper for veggie sweethearts or people with dairy hypersensitivities considering the way that most decisions contain milk.

Additionally, the Fuelings use different trimmings, so those with food hypersensitivities ought to scrutinize the names circumspectly.

Finally, the Optavia program isn't recommended for pregnant women since it can't meet their dietary needs.

May Brief Weight Recapture

Weight recoup may be a concern after you stop the program.

Directly, no assessment has reviewed weight regain after the Optavia diet. In light of everything, in an examination on a tantamount, 16-week Medifast diet, individuals recuperated an ordinary of 11 pounds (4.8 kg) inside 24 weeks of the fulfillment of the program.

One probably purpose behind weight recoup is your reliance on packaged food things. After the diet, it may be difficult to change to searching for and planning strong dinners.

Besides, due to the hair-raising calorie restriction of the 5&1 Plan, some weight regain may moreover be a direct result of an all the more moderate processing.

Optavia Fuelings Are Significantly Dealt With

The Optavia diet relies seriously upon prepackaged food things. In reality, you would eat 150 prepackaged Fuelings consistently on the 5&1 Plan.

This is a purpose behind concern; a similar number of these things are significantly arranged.

They contain a ton of food, included substances, sugar substitutes, and arranged vegetable oils, which may hurt your gut prosperity and add to steady irritation.

Carrageenan, a commonplace thickener and added substance used in various Fuelings, is gotten from red sea development. While research on its security is confined, animal and test-tube tests recommend that it may conversely impact stomach related prosperity and cause intestinal ulcers.

Moreover, various Fuelings contain maltodextrin, a thickening master that has been seemed to spike glucose levels and mischief your gut microorganisms.

While these additional substances are likely shielded in restricted amounts, using them a significant part of the time on the Optavia diet may assemble your threat of indications.

The program's guides are not prosperity specialists

Most Optavia guides have adequately shed pounds on the program anyway are not affirmed, prosperity specialists.

Hence, they are deficient in giving dietary or clinical urging. Henceforth, you should consider their bearing while at the same time mulling over different factors and speak with your human administration provider if you have any concerns.

In case you have a current prosperity condition, it's furthermore basic to advise a clinical provider or enrolled dietitian before starting another diet program.

Chapter IV: The Optavia Diet Guide

For a quick weight loss goal, the Optimal Weight 5&1 Plan may be the best plan to start with. Most people with the target of losing weight usually go for this plan as it helps them drop up to 12 pounds within 12 weeks.

In the Optimal Weight 5&1 Plan, you are expected to eat one lean and green meal and five OPTAVIA Fuelings. These meals are to be eaten every 2-3 hours intervals. Then, you will back it up with 30 minutes of exercise. Your coach will direct you on the best approach.

However, the daily carbs from meal and Fuelings should not exceed 100 grams. You can get meals and Fuelings from the company. Though it may not be cost-effective, this book is designed to help you save costs. You can prepare the meals by yourself to reduce costs.

There are many recipes in this book to help you along the process of your daily meals. You can also eat out, but keep in mind that you must follow the diet plan as instructed by your coach. However, alcohol is highly restricted for this plan.

Once you get to your desired weight, you are expected to enter the maintenance phase. This transition phase requires a gradual increase in your daily calorie intake to no more than 1,550 cal. You can add a wider variety of food to your daily meals, including fruits, whole grains, and low-fat dairy.

The maintenance phase is expected to last for 6 weeks before moving to the Optimal Health 3&3 Plan. Your daily food intake will be 3 OPTAVIA Fuelings and 3 lean and green meals in this plan.

In the OPTAVIA diet, most people that follow the diet usually opt for the 5&1 plan. The 5&1 program is made up of 5 Fuelings and 1 high protein low-carb meal. There are over 60 fueling options in the OPTAVIA diet, and these options include bars, puddings, shakes, soups, biscuits, etc. These Fuelings contain probiotics that help to promote digestive health.

The interesting aspect of the OPTAVIA diet is its flexibility, which makes it easier to work with. Once you reach your desired weight goal, you can easily switch to the 3&3 plan. Transitioning to this weight-maintenance plan is easy since you have already changed the old unhealthy eating habits. For those looking to consume more calories, the 4&2&1 plan is your best bet. With the 4&2&1 plan, you take 4 Fuelings, 2 healthy lean and green meals, and 1 snack.

How OPTAVIA Can Help You Lose Weight - Backed By Research

How much weight you lose on the OPTAVIA diet depends mostly on how active and how you follow the plan. If you stick with the plan and stay very active, you will lose more weight. Many have tried it, and it worked perfectly well. The following research studies show how effective the OPTAVIA diet can be when strictly followed. Though the research is mostly on Medifast, OPTAVIA and Medifast have identical macro-nutrients and can be interchanged to achieve the same result. So, the studies are valid for both OPTAVIA and Medifast plans.

- A study published in the Obesity journal in 2016 showed that after 12 weeks of observing the Medifast (OPTAVIA) diet guide, obese people lost 8.8% body weight.

- The study released by John Hopkins Medicine, which ran for 12 weeks, revealed that weight-loss programs like Medifast are effective for a long-term weight loss goal.

- A study in the Nutrition Journal in 2015 shows that 310 obese and overweight people who followed the Medifast (OPTAVIA) diet plan lost 24 lb in 12 weeks. In the 24th week, the average weight loss recorded was 35 lb.

- Another study published in the Nutrition Journal shows that 90 obese adults who followed the 5&1 plan lost an average of 30 pounds in 16 weeks.

- The analysis published in the Eating and Weight Disorder Journal in 2008 shows that average weight loss recorded on 324 obese patients in 12 weeks was 21 lb and 26 ½ lb after 24 weeks. However, these patients also took appetite suppressant.

Is OPTAVIA Diet Easy To Follow?

If you are someone like me that likes trying so many treats and yummy recipes almost every day, the OPTAVIA diet may not be easy in the long term. However, the OPTAVIA diet is programmed to accommodate both long-term and short-term goals. There are three major diet plans to choose from to suit your desired eating habit.

The 5&1 plan may not be easy in the long-term, but there are over 60 fueling options to work with. Moreover, you have many resources where you can get recipes, including this cookbook with so many mouthwatering recipes to make.

Unlike most weight-loss diets, you don't need to stress yourself counting calories, points, or carbs. Though they are needed for reference purposes, you don't need to kill yourself over it as long as the meals you are taking are OPTAVIA-compliance lean and green meals.

Interestingly, you can easily eat out while on the OPTAVIA diet. The main thing is for you to understand the guidelines and follow them judiciously. You can download the eating out the guide from the company website to help you easily navigate the buffets and eateries.

How Much Exercise Is Needed?

Like we stated earlier, if you want to lose weight as desired, you need to be active. Exercise helps you achieve that. Find the right exercise you can easily do daily and incorporate it into your plan.

OPTAVIA highly recommends at least 30 minutes of exercise almost every day. If it's walking, walk. If it requires doing some minor workouts, do them and enjoy the process. Remember, happiness is of the utmost importance in your daily life. So, engage in exercise that you enjoy most and are super healthy for you. Don't overstress your body, don't go overboard. You can get recommendations from your doctor or coach if you have any.

Health Risks Of OPTAVIA Diet

Though there is no noteworthy risk(s) associated with the OPTAVIA diet, we should not conclude that it is completely safe for everyone. Anyone on any diet is usually advised to watch out for side effects and stop the diet if any health-threatening effect surfaces. Some possible side effects to consider include but are not limited to bad breath, loss of hair, headache, loose skin, constipation, dizziness, menstrual cycle change, diarrhea, cramps, etc.

Moreover, research has shown that low-calorie diets may pose a high risk of health complications such as gallstone.

Pregnant women and nursing mothers are not advised to be on this plan unless recommended by your health specialist. If you are younger than 13, this diet plan may not be safe for you. Discuss with your doctor first before using the plan for your weight loss goal. The same suggestion applies to those with liver disease, cancer, or kidney disease.

Are you on medication? This includes lithium, diabetes medication, and warfarin. Even high blood medication is not an exception. Discuss with your health specialist first before engaging in the diet.

These suggestions don't mean that OPTAVIA is not healthy or safe. These are mere suggestions that go beyond the OPTAVIA diet. This group of people is usually advised to discuss with their doctors before using any form of low-calorie diet program, which OPTAVIA happens to be one of them.

Can OPTAVIA Reverse Heart Disease? Research Suggestions

According to the Food and Drug Administration, high-quality soy protein promotes heart health. OPTAVIA Fuelings are said to contain high-quality soy protein in enough amounts to promote heart health.

However, the OPTAVIA diet may not be the best diet for heart health, but it contains a very low amount of fat and cholesterol, which is good for preventing and controlling heart diseases. Moreover, some studies suggest that the OPTAVIA diet, since it has the same macronutrients as Medifast, may promote heart health.

- The study in 2017 sponsored by Medifast, which is published in Nutrition and Diet Journal, shows that the Medifast (OPTAVIA) diet may significantly lower blood pressure.

- The study carried out by Medifast in 2015 shows that the 4&2&1 diet plan can significantly improve dieters' blood pressure.

• In 2010, another study published in the Nutrition Journal shows that the diet helped to decline pulse rate, blood pressure, and the blood levels of the marker (C-reactive Protein) of inflammation, which predicts the risk of heart disease. The same study revealed a 4-inch reduction in the waist size of participants with abnormal waist size and fat that could indicate heart disease risk.

Can OPTAVIA Prevent And Reverse Diabetes?

Though reserve has not shown any advantage OPTAVIA has over other diets regarding this issue, it is apparent that OPTAVIA may help prevent and control diabetes.

Obesity and overweight are among the risk factors for type 2 diabetes. This simply means that OPTAVIA could control and prevent type 2 diabetes since it is very effective for weight loss.

A study carried out in 2017 and published in Nutrition Journal shows that OPTAVIA can help diabetics lose body fat, lower pulse, blood pressure, and waist size.

The Diabetes Educator study showed that Medifast (OPTAVIA) could help improve blood sugar and insulin levels.

Which Diet Is Compatible With OPTAVIA?

Some diets can be incorporated into the OPTAVIA plan. These diets include vegetarian, gluten-free, and low-salt. Vegan, keto, and Dr. Sebi's diet may not work with OPTAVIA.

Best Foods For OPTAVIA Diet

Your homemade meals are expected to be mostly low-carb vegetables, lean proteins, and a few healthy fats. Low-carb beverages such as coffee, water, tea, unsweetened almond milk, etc. are allowed, but in small amounts.

The recommended foods for your lean and green meals are;

- Fish and Shellfish: trout, halibut, salmon, shrimp, tuna, crab, lobster, scallops.
- Meat: Lean beef, pork chop, tenderloin, turkey, chicken, lamb.

• Eggs: egg whites, whole eggs, and egg beaters.

• Soy: tofu

• Oil: vegetable oils - flaxseed, olive, canola, walnut, lemon oil, etc

• Fats: avocado, olives, almonds, pistachios, reduced-fat margarine, walnuts, etc.

• Vegetables: zucchini, cauliflower, celery, mushrooms, eggplant, pepper, spinach, cucumbers, squash, broccoli, collard, jicama, etc.

• Snacks (sugar-free): mints, popsicle, gum, gelatin, etc.

• Beverages (sugar-free): coffee, water, tea, almond milk, etc.

• Seasoning and condiments: spices, dried herbs, salsa, cocktail sauce, yellow mustard, lemon juice, soy sauce, lime juice, etc.

Avoid These Foods

Except for the Fuelings carbs, the OPTAVIA diet restricts most foods and beverages with carb content. Some fats are not allowed, including fried foods. Avoid the following foods in your daily meals;

• Refined grains: including pasta, flour tortillas, cookies, white rice, white bread, cakes, biscuits, etc.

• Whole fat dairy: including yogurt, milk, and cheese.

• Fried foods: including fish, veggies, meats, pastries, etc.

• Fats: like coconut oil, butter, etc.

• Alcohol: all types.

• Beverages: like an energy drink, fruit juice, sweet tea, soda, etc

If you are on the 5&1 plan, you need to avoid the following foods in your daily meal. You can introduce them in the transition phase;

• Starchy veggies: white potatoes, sweet potatoes, peas, and corn.

• Whole grains: brown rice, whole grain bread, whole-wheat pasta, etc.

• Low-fat dairy: cheese, yogurt, and milk.

• Legumes: beans, peas, soybeans, lentils, etc.

• Fruits: fresh fruits. Eat more berries when you enter the transition phase.

Chapter V: More info about Optavia Diet

Discussion with a mentor to help figure out which Optavia plan to follow, set weight reduction objectives, and acclimate yourself with the program withstanding the arrangement you pick; you start by having a telephone

Beginning Stages

For weight reduction, the vast majority start with the Optimal Weight 5&1 Plan. An 800–1,000 calorie routine said to assist you with dropping 12 pounds (5.4 kg) for more than 12 weeks.

On this arrangement, you eat 5 Optavia Fuelings and 1 Lean and Green supper every day. You're intended to eat one supper each 2–3 hours and fuse 30 minutes of moderate exercise most days of the week.

Altogether, the fuelings and feast give close to 100 grams of carbs every day. You request these suppers from your mentor's site, as Optavia mentors get paid on commission.

Lean and Green suppers are intended to be high in protein and low in carbs. One dinner offers 5–7 ounces (145–200 grams) of cooked lean protein, three servings of non-dull vegetables, and up to 2 servings of solid fats. This arrangement additionally incorporates one discretionary nibble for each day, which must be endorsed by your mentor. Plan-endorsed snacks include three celery sticks, 1/2 cup (60 grams) of without sugar gelatin, or 1/2 ounce (14 grams) of nuts.

The program likewise incorporates feasting out guides that disclose how to arrange a Lean and Green supper with your preferred coffee. Remember that liquor is firmly disheartened on the 5&1 Plan.

Support Stage

When you arrive at your ideal weight, you enter a 6-week change stage, which includes gradually expanding calories to close to 1,550 calories for each day and mixing it up of foods, including entire grains, organic products, and low-fat dairy.

Following a month and a half, you're intended to move onto the Optimal Health 3&3 Plan, which incorporates 3 Lean and Green dinners and 3 Fuelings every day, in addition to proceeded Optavia training.

The individuals who experience supported accomplishment on the program have the choice to get prepared as an Optavia mentor.

Would Optavia Diet Help You With Shedding Pounds?

The Optavia diet is intended to help individuals get thinner and fat by diminishing calories and carbs through part-controlled dinners and tidbits.

The 5&1 arrangement limits calories to 800–1,000 calories each day partitioned between 6 divided controlled meals.

While the examination is blended, a few investigations have indicated more prominent weight reduction with full or halfway meal supplanting plans contrasted and customary calorie-confined eating regimens.

Studies likewise uncover that lessening by and massive calorie admission is viable for weight and fat misfortune—as are low carb, at any rate, temporarily.

A 16-week concentration in 198 individuals with abundant weight or stoutness found that those on Optavia's 5&1 Plan had fundamentally lower weight, fat levels, abdomen periphery, contrasted, and benchmark group.

With 28.1% of members losing over 10%. It may recommend extra advantages, as research partners reduce weight by 5–10% with a diminished danger of coronary illness and type 2 diabetes.

The one-on-one instructing might be useful too.

A similar report found that people on the 5&1 eating regimen who finished in any event 75% of the training meetings lost more than twice as much weight as the individuals who partook in fewer meetings.

No different, a few various examinations exhibit a massive improvement in short-and long-haul weight reduction and diet adherence in programs that incorporate progressing training.

Presently, no examinations have analyzed the drawn-out aftereffects of the Optavia diet. An analysis of a comparative Medifast plan noticed that solitary 25% of members kept up the eating routine for as long as one year.

Another test gave some weight to recover during the weight support stage following the 5&1 Medifast diet.

The main contrast between the 5&1 Medifast diet and the 5&1 Optavia Plan is that Optavia incorporates instructing.

In general, more research is expected to survey the Optavia diet's drawn-out viability.

Other Potential Advantages

The Optavia diet has extra advantages that may support weight reduction and by and large health.

Simple to follow

As the eating routine generally depends on prepackaged Fuelings, you're just answerable for preparing one feast every day on the 5&1 Plan.

Besides, each arrangement accompanies supper logs, and test dinner intends to make it simpler to follow.

While you're urged to cook 1–3 Lean and Green dinners every day, contingent upon the arrangement, they're easy to make—as the program incorporates detailed plans and a rundown of food choices.

Besides, the individuals who aren't interested in preparing meals can purchase dinner packages called Flavors of Homes.

May improve circulatory strain

Optavia projects may help improve circulatory strain through weight reduction and restricted sodium admission.

While the Optavia diet has not been explicitly investigated, a 40-week study of 90 overweight people in a comparable Medifast program revealed a decrease in blood pressure.

Also, all Optavia dinner plans are intended to give under 2,300 mg of sodium for each day—even though it's dependent upon you to pick low sodium choices for Lean and Green suppers.

That is because higher sodium admission is connected to an expanded danger of hypertension and coronary illness in salt-touchy people.

Offers progressing support

Optavia's health mentors are accessible all through weight reduction and upkeep programs.

As noted above, one examination found a massive connection between the number of training meetings on the Optavia 5&1 Plan and improved weight reduction.

Moreover, this plan suggests that having a mentor or advisor may help in the long-run.

Chapter VI: Recipes for breakfast

This list of some excellent recipes is very useful for the Optavia diet, with related preparations and nutritional values.

1. Protein Oatcakes

Preparation Time: 10 minutes

Cooking Time: 5 minutes

Servings: 1

INGREDIENTS:

70g oatmeal

15g protein

1 egg white

½ cup of water

½ teaspoon cinnamon

60g curd

1 teaspoon cacao powder

15g sugar

DIRECTIONS:

1. Mix the oatmeal, protein, egg white, and water in a bowl.
2. Preheat a saucepan to medium heat.
3. Place the mixture into the saucepan.
4. While waiting, prepare the topping by mixing the curd, cinnamon, and sugar in a second bowl.
5. Remove the oatcake from the saucepan when it becomes golden-brown.
6. Serve on a plate.
7. Add the topping and cocoa powder.

NUTRITION:

Calories: 440

Protein: 1.1g

Fiber: 0.8g

Carbohydrates: 6.1g

2. Orange Ricotta Pancakes

Preparation Time: 10 minutes

Cooking Time: 5 minutes

Servings: 1

INGREDIENTS:

¾ cup all-purpose flour

½ tablespoon baking powder

2 teaspoons sugar

½ teaspoon salt

3 separated eggs

1 cup fresh ricotta

¾ cup whole milk

½ teaspoon pure vanilla extract

1 large ripe orange

DIRECTIONS:

1. Mix the flour, baking powder, sugar in a large bowl.

2. Add a pinch of salt.

3. In a separate bowl, whisk egg yolk, ricotta, milk, orange zest, and orange juice.

4. Add some vanilla extract for additional flavor.

5. Followed by the dry ingredients to the ricotta mixture and mix adequately.

6. Stir the egg white in a different bowl, and then gently fold it in the ricotta mixture.

7. Preheat saucepan to medium heat and brush with some butter until evenly spread.

8. Use a measuring cup to drop the batter onto the saucepan, ensure the pan is not crowded.

9. Allow cooking for 2 minutes.

10. Flip the food when you notice the edges begin to set, and bubbles form in the center.

11. Cook the meat for another 1 to 2 minutes.

12. Serve with any toppings of your choice.

NUTRITION:

Calories: 160

Fat: 10g

Carbohydrate: 28g

Protein: 6g

3. Asian Scrambled Egg

Preparation Time: 10 minutes

Cooking Time: 10 minutes

Servings: 1

INGREDIENTS:

1 large egg

1/2 teaspoons light soy sauce

1/8 teaspoon white pepper

1 tablespoon vegetable oil

DIRECTIONS:

1. Beat the eggs in a bowl.

2. To the beaten egg, add soy sauce, one teaspoon vegetable oil, and pepper.

3. Preheat a saucepan on high heat.

4. Add the two tablespoons oil to the saucepan.

5. Then add the mixture of the beaten egg.

6. The edges will begin to cook.

7. Lessen the heat to medium and carefully scramble the eggs.

8. Turn off heat and transfer into a bowl.

9. Serve hot and enjoy

NUTRITION:

Calories: 200

Fat: 6.7g

Protein: 6.1g

Carbohydrates: 1g

4. Artichoke Frittatas

Preparation Time: 10 minutes

Cooking Time: 30 minutes

Servings: 1

INGREDIENTS:

2.5 oz. dry spinach

1/4 red bell pepper

Artichoke (drain the liquid)

Green onions

Dried tomatoes

Two eggs

Italian seasoning

Salt

Pepper

DIRECTIONS:

1. Preheat oven to medium heat.

2. Brush a bit of oil on the cast-iron skillet.

3. Mix all the vegetables.

4. Add some seasoning.

5. Spread the vegetables evenly in the pan.

6. Whisk the eggs and add some milk.

7. Add some salt and pepper.

8. Mix in some cheese (helps to make it fluffier).

9. Pour the egg mixture into the saucepan.

10. Place the pan inside the oven for about 30 minutes.

11. Enjoy!

NUTRITION:

Calories: 160

Protein: 7g

Carbohydrates: 4g

Fat: 3.5g

5. Chocolate Sweet Potato Pudding

Preparation Time: 5 minutes

Cooking Time: 2 minutes

Servings: 1

INGREDIENTS:

2 well-cooked sweet potatoes

2 tablespoons cocoa powder

2 tablespoons maple syrup

¼ cups plant-based milk (for example, almond milk)

¼ tablespoons salt

¼ tablespoons vanilla extract

DIRECTIONS:

1. Inside the food processor, put all the ingredients.

2. Blend thoroughly for about 30 seconds to 1 minute.

3. Voilà!

NUTRITION:

Calories: 200

Fat: 1.5g

Carbohydrates: 23.4g

Fiber: 1.3g

6. Peanut Butter and Protein Pancake

Preparation Time: 10 minutes

Cooking Time: 15 minutes

Servings: 1

INGREDIENTS:

½ cup oat flour

½ cup gluten-free chocolate pancake mix ½ cup almond milk

1 egg

1 tablespoon coconut water

1 tablespoon peanut butter

Fresh fruits slices

DIRECTIONS:

1. Preheat a saucepan to medium heat.

2. Mix the flour and the pancake mix in a mixing bowl.

3. Mix the almond milk and eggs with coconut water in another bowl.

4. Mix the dry and wet ingredients thoroughly to form a delicate batter.

5. Spray the preheated saucepan with some coconut oil.

6. Put the batter into the saucepan with a measuring cup and allow it to cook for a few minutes.

7. Allow to cool and top with peanut butter and fresh fruit slices.

NUTRITION:

Calories: 380

Protein: 22g

Carbohydrates: 16g

7. Zucchini Frittata

Preparation Time: 20 minutes

Cooking Time: 20 minutes

Servings: 1

INGREDIENTS:

2 large zucchinis

1½ teaspoon of salt

2 eggs

½ cup chopped green onions

1 cup flour

½ teaspoon of black pepper

1 teaspoon of baking powder

2 tablespoons of oil

DIRECTIONS:

1. Wash the two zucchinis.

2. Cut off the zucchinis on its ends and grate them in a large mixing bowl.

3. Stir in 1 teaspoon of salt and set aside for about 10 minutes (The salt helps draw out the water from the zucchinis).

4. Squeeze dry the grated zucchinis to remove as much water as possible.

5. Then followed by the two whole eggs and the chopped green onions.

6. In a bowl, mix a cup flour, ½ teaspoon of salt, ½ teaspoon of black pepper, and one teaspoon of baking powder.

7. Next, pour the smaller bowl contents into those of the larger bowl containing the grated zucchinis.

8. Stir them all together and make sure they are well mixed.

9. Preheat a saucepan to medium temperature and add two tablespoons of oil.

10. Add the zucchini mixture a heaping tablespoonful at a time.

11. Sauté the mixture for about 4 minutes on each side to achieve a golden-brown color.

12. Add more oil to the pan if needed.

13. Serve and enjoy!

NUTRITION:

Calories: 200

Protein: 7g

Carbohydrates: 4g

Fat: 3.5g

8. Tex-Mex Tofu Breakfast Tacos

Preparation Time: 10 minutes

Cooking Time: 15 minutes

Servings: 1

INGREDIENTS:

8 oz. firm tofu

1 cup well-cooked black bean

1/4 red onion

1 cup fresh coriander

1 ripe avocado

1/2 cup salsa

1 medium-sized lime

5 whole corn tortillas

1/2 teaspoon garlic powder

1/2 teaspoon chili powder

1/8 teaspoon of sea salt

1 tablespoon salsa

1 tablespoon water

DIRECTIONS:

1. Dice the red onions, avocados, coriander, and keep in separate bowls.

2. Also, slice the limes and keep in individual bowls.

3. In a clean towel. Wrap the tofu and place under a cast-iron skillet.

4. In the meantime, heat a saucepan to medium heat.

5. Cook the black beans in the saucepan and add a little salt, cumin, and chili powder.

6. Then decrease the heat to a low simmer and set aside.

7. Add the tofu spices and salsa into a bowl, then add some water and set aside.

8. Heat another skillet to medium heat.

9. Pour some oil into the skillet, and then crumble the tofu into it.

10. Stir-fry for about 5 minutes until the tofu begins to brown.

11. Add some seasoning and continue to cook for about 5 to 10 minutes and then set aside.

12. Heat the tortillas in the oven to 250°F.

13. Top the tortillas with tofu scramble, avocado, salsa, coriander, black beans, and lime juice.

14. Serve immediately.

NUTRITION:

Calories: 350

Fat: 6.5g

Carbohydrates: 23.6g

Protein: 21.5g

9. Mocha Oatmeal

Preparation Time: 5 minutes

Cooking Time: 10 minutes

Servings: 1

INGREDIENTS:

1 banana

½ cup oats

1 cup coffee

¼ teaspoon salt

1 teaspoon walnut

½ teaspoon cacao powder

1 cup milk

Honey

DIRECTIONS:

1. Preheat a saucepan to medium heat.

2. Put the oats in a saucepan.

3. Slice the banana, mash them, and add them to the oats.

4. Add coffee, walnuts, cacao powder, and salt.

5. Stir, and you may want to wait for it to simmer, practically until the mixture becomes sticky inconsistency.

6. Serve in a bowl and add milk and honey as desired.

7. Enjoy!

NUTRITION:

Calories: 400

Carbohydrates: 51g

Fats: 5g

Fiber: 8g

10. Black and Blueberry Protein Smoothie

Preparation Time: 5 minutes

Cooking Time: 0 minutes

Servings: 1

INGREDIENTS:

1 cup sugar-free coconut milk (or any other plant-based milk of your choice)

1 scoop vanilla or natural protein powder

6 oz. fat-free vanilla Greek yogurt

2 tablespoons of milled flaxseed

1 cup berries (black or blue)

1 cup ice

DIRECTIONS:

1. In the food processor, place all the ingredients.

2. Blend until smooth.

3. Pour into a cup and enjoy it.

NUTRITION:

Calories: 360

Fats: 1.5g

Protein: 49g

Carbohydrates: 40g

11. Shake Cake Fueling

Preparation Time: 5 minutes

Cooking Time: 0 minutes

Servings: 1

INGREDIENTS:

1 packet optavia shakes.

¼ teaspoon baking powder

2 tablespoons eggbeaters or egg whites

2 tablespoons water.

Other options that are not compulsory include sweetener, reduced-fat cream cheese, ketchup

DIRECTIONS:

1. Begin by preheating the oven.

2. Mix all the ingredients; begin with the dry ingredients first before adding the wet ingredients.

3. After the mixture/batter is ready, pour gently into muffin cups.

4. Inside the oven, place, and bake for about 16–18minutes or until it is baked and ready. Allow it to cool completely.

5. Add additional toppings of your choice and ensure your delicious shake cake is refreshing.

NUTRITION:

Calories: 896

Fat: 37g

Carbohydrate: 115g

Protein: 34g

12. Cauliflower Crust Pizza

Preparation Time: 15 minutes

Cooking Time: 30–35 minutes

Servings: 1

INGREDIENTS:

1/4 cauliflower (it should be cut into smaller portions)

1/16 grated parmesan cheese

1/2 egg

½ teaspoon Italian seasoning

1/16 teaspoon kosher salt

1 cups of freshly grated mozzarella

1/4 cup spicy pizza sauce.

Basil leaves, for garnishing.

DIRECTIONS:

1. Begin by preheating your oven while using the parchment paper to rim the baking sheet.

2. Process the cauliflower into a fine powder and then transfer to a bowl before putting it into the microwave. Leave for about 5–6 minutes to get it soft.

3. Transfer the microwaved cauliflower to a clean and dry kitchen towel. Leave it to cool.

4. When cold, use the kitchen towel to wrap the cauliflower and then get rid of all the moisture by wringing the towel. Continue squeezing until water is gone completely.

5. Put the cauliflower, Italian seasoning, parmesan, egg, salt, and mozzarella (1 cup). Stir very well until well combined.

6. Transfer the combined mixture to the baking sheet previously prepared, pressing it into a 10-inch round shape.

7. Wait for it to bake until it becomes golden in color.

8. Take the baked crust out of the oven and use the spicy pizza sauce

and mozzarella (the leftover 1 cup) to top it. Put it again inside the oven for ten more minutes until the cheese melts and looks bubbly.

9. Garnish using fresh basil leaves. You can also enjoy this with salad.

NUTRITION:

Calories: 230

Fat: 8g

Carbohydrate: 28g

Protein: 6g

13. Zucchini Fritters

Preparation Time: 5 minutes

Cooking Time: 15 minutes

Servings: 1

INGREDIENTS:

1/4 pound grated zucchini

1/4 teaspoon salt

1/16 cup grated parmesan

1/16 cup flour

1/2 cloves minced garlic

1/2 tablespoon olive oil

1/4 large egg

Newly ground black pepper and kosher salt to taste

DIRECTIONS:

1. Put the grated zucchini into a colander over the sink.

2. Add your salt and toss it to mix properly, then leave it to settle for about 10 minutes.

3. Next, use a clean cheesecloth to drain the zucchini completely.

4. Combine drained zucchini, parmesan, garlic, flour, and the beaten egg in a large bowl, mix, and season with pepper and salt.

5. Then, pour the olive oil into a skillet applying medium-high heat.

6. Use a tablespoon to scoop batter for each cake, put in the oil, and flatten using a spatula.

7. Allow to cook until the underside is richly golden brown, then flip over to the other side and cook.

8. Your delicious zucchini fritters are ready to be served.

NUTRITION:

Calories: 105.1

Fat: 2.8g

Carbohydrate: 15.8g

Protein: 6g

14. Optavia Pizza Hack

Preparation Time: 5–10 minutes

Cooking Time: 15–20 minutes

Servings: 1

INGREDIENTS:

1/4 fueling garlic mashed potato

1/2 egg whites

1/4 tablespoon baking powder

3/4 oz. reduced-fat shredded mozzarella

1/8 cup sliced white mushrooms

1/16 cup pizza sauce

3/4 oz. ground beef

1/4 sliced black olives

You also need a sauté pan, baking sheets, and parchment paper

DIRECTIONS:

1. Start by preheating the oven to 400°F.

2. Mix your baking powder and garlic potato packet.

3. Add egg whites to your mixture and stir well until it blends.

4. Line the baking sheet with parchment paper and pour the mixed batter onto it.

5. Put another parchment paper on top of the batter and spread it to a 1/8-inch circle.

6. Then place another baking sheet on top; this way, the matter is between two baking sheets.

7. Place into an oven and bake for about 8 minutes until the pizza crust is golden brown.

8. For the toppings, place your ground beef in a sauté pan and fry until it's brown, and wash your mushrooms very well.

9. After the crust is baked, remove the top layer of parchment paper carefully to prevent the paper from sticking to the pizza crust.

10. Put your toppings on top of the crust and bake for an extra 8 minutes.

11. Once ready, slide the pizza off the parchment paper and into a plate.

NUTRITION:

Calories: 478

Protein: 30g

Carbohydrates: 22g

Fats: 29g

15. Optavia Biscuit Pizza

Preparation Time: 5 minutes

Cooking Time: 15–20 minutes

Servings: 1

INGREDIENTS:

1/4 sachet optavia buttermilk cheddar and herb biscuit

1/4 tablespoon tomato sauce

1/4 tablespoon low-fat shredded cheese

1/4 table of water

Parchment paper

DIRECTIONS:

1. You may begin by preheating the oven to about 350°F.

2. Mix the biscuit and water and stir properly.

3. In the parchment paper, pour the mixture and spread it into a thin circle. Allow cooking for 10 minutes.

4. Take it out and add the tomato sauce and shredded cheese.

5. Bake it for a few more minutes.

NUTRITION:

Calories: 478

Protein: 30g

Carbohydrates: 22g

Fats: 29g

16. Mini Mac in a Bowl

Preparation Time: 5 minutes

Cooking Time: 15 minutes

Servings: 1

INGREDIENTS:

5 oz. lean ground beef

2 tablespoons diced white or yellow onion.

1/8 teaspoon onion powder

1/8 teaspoon white vinegar

1 oz. dill pickle slices

1 teaspoon sesame seed

3 cups shredded romaine lettuce

Cooking spray

2 tablespoons reduced-fat shredded cheddar cheese

2 tablespoons wish-bone light thousand islands as dressing

DIRECTIONS:

1. Place a lightly greased small skillet on fire to heat.

2. Add your onion to cook for about 2–3 minutes.

3. Next, add the beef and allow it to cook until it is brown.

4. Next, mix your vinegar and onion powder with the dressing.

5. Finally, top the lettuce with the cooked meat and sprinkle cheese on it; add your pickle slices.

6. Drizzle the mixture with the sauce and sprinkle the sesame seeds also.

7. Your mini mac in a bowl is ready for consumption.

NUTRITION:

Calories: 150

Protein: 21g

Carbohydrates: 32g

Fats: 19g

17. Lean and Green Smoothie 1

Preparation Time: 5 minutes

Cooking Time: 0 minutes

Servings: 1

INGREDIENTS:

2 ½ cups of kale leaves

¾ cup chilled apple juice

1 cup cubed pineapple

½ cup frozen green grapes

½ cup chopped apple

DIRECTIONS:

1. Place the pineapple, apple juice, apple, frozen seedless grapes, and kale leaves in a blender.

2. Cover and blend until it's smooth.

3. Smoothie is ready and can be garnished with halved grapes if you wish.

NUTRITION:

Calories: 81

Protein: 2g

Carbohydrates: 19g

Fats: 1g

18. Lean and Green Smoothie 2

Preparation Time: 5 minutes

Cooking Time: 0 minutes

Servings: 1

INGREDIENTS:

6 kale leaves

2 peeled oranges

2 cups mango kombucha

2 cups chopped pineapple

2 cups of water

DIRECTIONS:

1. Break up the oranges, place in the blender.

2. Add the mango kombucha, chopped pineapple, and kale leaves into the blender.

3. Blend everything until it is smooth.

4. Smoothie is ready to be taken.

NUTRITION:

Calories: 81

Protein: 2g

Carbohydrates: 19g

Fats: 1g

19. Lean and Green Chicken Pesto Pasta

Preparation Time: 5 minutes

Cooking Time: 15 minutes

Servings: 1

INGREDIENTS:

3 cups raw kale leaves

2 tablespoon olive oil

2 cups fresh basil

¼ teaspoon salt

3 tablespoon lemon juice

3 garlic cloves

2 cups cooked chicken breast

1 cup baby spinach

6 oz. uncooked chicken pasta

3 oz. diced fresh mozzarella

Basil leaves or red pepper flakes to garnish

DIRECTIONS:

1. Start by making the pesto, add the kale, lemon juice, basil, garlic cloves, olive oil, and salt to a blender and blend until it is smooth.

2. Add pepper to taste.

3. Cook the pasta and strain off the water. Reserve ¼ cup of the liquid.

4. Get a bowl and mix everything, the cooked pasta, pesto, diced chicken, spinach, mozzarella, and the reserved pasta liquid.

5. Sprinkle the mixture with additional chopped basil or red paper flakes (optional).

6. Now, your salad is ready. You may serve it warm or chilled. Also, it can be taken as a salad mix-ins or as a side dish. Leftovers should be stored in the refrigerator inside an air-tight container for 3–5 days.

NUTRITION:

Calories: 244

Protein: 20.5g

Carbohydrates: 22.5g

Fats: 10g

20. Tropical Greens Smoothie

Preparation Time: 5 Minutes

Cooking Time: 0 Minutes

Servings: 1

INGREDIENTS:

1 banana

1/2 large navel orange, peeled and segmented 1/2 cup frozen mango chunks

1 cup frozen spinach

1 celery stalk, broken into pieces

1 tablespoon cashew butter or almond butter 1/2 tablespoon spiraling

1/2 tablespoon ground flaxseed

1/2 cup unsweetened nondairy milk

Water, for thinning (optional)

DIRECTIONS:

1. In a high-speed blender or food processor, combine the bananas, orange, mango, spinach, celery, cashew butter, spiraling (if using), flaxseed, and milk.

2. Blend until creamy, adding more milk or water to thin the smoothie if too thick. Serve immediately—it is best served fresh.

NUTRITION:

Calories: 391

Fat: 12g

Protein: 13g

Carbohydrates: 68g

Fiber: 13g

21. Vitamin C Smoothie Cubes

Preparation Time: 5 minutes

Cooking Time: 8 hours to chill

Servings: 1

INGREDIENTS:

1/8 large papaya

1/8 mango

1/4 cups chopped pineapple, fresh or frozen

1/8 cup raw cauliflower florets, fresh or frozen

1/4 large navel oranges, peeled and halved

1/4 large orange bell pepper stemmed, seeded, and coarsely chopped

DIRECTIONS:

1. Halve the papaya and mango, remove the pits, and scoop their soft flesh into a high-speed blender.

2. Add the pineapple, cauliflower, oranges, and bell pepper. Blend until smooth.

3. Evenly divide the puree between 2 (16-compartment) ice cube trays and place them on a level surface in your freezer. Freeze for at least 8 hours.

4. The cubes can be left in the ice cube trays until use or transferred to a freezer bag. The frozen cubes are good for about three weeks in a standard freezer or up to 6 months in a chest freezer.

NUTRITION:

Calories: 96

Fat: 1g

Protein: 2g

Carbohydrates: 24g

Fiber: 4g

22. Overnight Chocolate Chia Pudding

Preparation Time: 2 minutes

Cooking Time: Overnight to Chill

Servings: 1

INGREDIENTS:

1/8 cup chia seeds

1/2 cup unsweetened nondairy milk

1 tablespoon raw cacao powder

1/2 teaspoon vanilla extract

1/2 teaspoon pure maple syrup

DIRECTIONS:

1. Stir together the chia seeds, milk, cacao powder, vanilla, and maple syrup in a large bowl. Divide between 2 (½-pint) covered glass jars or containers. Refrigerate overnight.

2. Stir before serving.

NUTRITION:

Calories: 213

Fat: 10g

Protein: 9g

Carbohydrates: 20g

Fiber: 15g

Chapter VIII: Snack food

The dishes in this section are genuinely healthy and satisfying, unlike other snacks and party foods. This means two things: one, whether you serve one or two of these foods before dinner, you may choose to cut down on amounts at the meal itself, and two, you may also be able to use many of these dishes as light meals and on your own. This is an incredibly useful idea-just set out a large tray of cut up veggies and dip, some wings, and a bowl of nut mix for family movie night and call it supper.

23. Addictive Wings

You'll understand the title if you try them. They're absolutely, entirely irresistible! These are a little sticky and time-consuming to produce, but every second is worth it. They're going to confuse the hell out of your mates too, and you're going to wish you made some more of them. The very next day, they taste amazing too.

Preparation Time: 30 min

Cooking Time: 1 hour

INGREDIENTS:

8 pounds of chicken wings

cup grated Parmesan cheese

tablespoons dried parsley

2 tablespoon dried oregano

A teaspoons paprika

2 teaspoon salt

1 teaspoon pepper

1 cup butter

DIRECTIONS:

1. Preheat your oven to about 350 ° F.

2. Break the wings into drumsticks and save the ends.

3. In a cup, mix the Parmesan cheese with the oregano, parsley, paprika, salt, and pepper.

4. Using foil to line a wide baking pan. (Do not miss this stage, or a week later, you'll still be cleaning the pan.)

5. In a small bowl or tub, melt the butter.

6. Dip each drumstick in butter first, roll in the mixture of cheese and seasoning, and place it in a foil-lined saucepan.

7. Bake for about 1 hour and then hit yourself for not getting a double recipe created!

NUTRITION:

About 70 pieces, each with only a trace of carbohydrates, a trace of fiber, and 6 grams of protein.

24. Peanut Wings

Try making these if you enjoy Chinese barbecued spareribs.

Preparation Time: 1 hour

Cooking Time: 1 hour

INGREDIENTS:

2/4 cup soy sauce

6 tablespoons natural peanut butter

4 tablespoons dry sherry

tablespoon oil

tablespoon apple cider vinegar

A teaspoons Chinese Five Spice powder

2/4 teaspoon red pepper flakes (or more, if you want them hotter)

2 clove garlic, crushed

24 chicken wings or 36 drumsticks

DIRECTIONS:

1. Oven preheats to 325 °F.

2. In a food processor or blender, place the Splendor, soy sauce, peanut butter, oil, sherry, vinegar, pepper flakes, seasoning powder, and garlic combine well.

3. If you've got whole wings of chicken and you want to turn them into drumsticks, do it now. (This is preferential and not crucial.)

4. Assemble the wings in a wide baking pan and spill over them the mixed sauce, then flip over and cover them on both sides.

5. Let them stay (an hour is much better) for at least half an hour.

6. Bake the wings for an hour, rotating when baking every 20 minutes.

7. Place them on a serving platter when the wings are finished, and scrub the sauce from the pan back into the food processor or blender. Blend once more to make it seamless for just a second, and serve with the wings.

NUTRITION:

36 pieces, each with 1 gram of carbohydrates, a trace of fiber, and 5 grams of protein.

25. Hot Wings

Using store-bought Buffalo Wing sauce instead of a combination of dry spices, you'd like to improve it. The bulk of wing sauces has no sugar in them and is very low in carbohydrates.

Preparation Time: 15 min

Cooking Time: 50 min

INGREDIENTS:

4 pounds of chicken wings, cut into drumsticks

4 teaspoons of dried thyme

4 teaspoons of paprika

A teaspoon of curry powder

A teaspoon of dried oregano

2 teaspoon of cayenne pepper

DIRECTIONS:

1. Preheat your oven to about 375 ° F.

2. In a cup, mix the cinnamon, curry, oregano, paprika, and thyme well.

3. Assemble the wings in a large baking pan and thinly spray the mixture over them, rotating on both sides to cover.

4. For 45 to 50 minutes to bake, or until crispy. Serve ranch or goat cheese dressing and celery sticks with conventional side dishes, if needed.

NUTRITION:

About 36 pieces, each with a trace of carbohydrates, a trace of fiber, and 4 grams of protein.

26. Pepper & Paprika Wings

These wings are easy to make, and they get ready in less than an hour, which makes them an excellent party snack.

Preparation Time: 10 min

Cooking Time: 50 min

INGREDIENTS:

Paprika

Pepper to your taste

Salt to your taste

4 cloves garlic, crushed

6 tablespoons of olive oil

40 chicken wing drumsticks

DIRECTIONS:

1. Preheat your oven to about 350 ° F.

2. Assemble the wings in a baking tray so they do not touch each other.

3. Mix the oil and garlic in a bowl and brush it over the wings using a spoon. Made sure that you do get some crushed garlic over each bit.

4. Dab the wings with some salt and pepper to taste, then dust with just enough paprika to make them all reddish.

5. Roast for 15 to 20 minutes; switch sides and season with salt, pepper, and paprika on the other side.

6. Roast for another 30 minutes, turning around every 15 to 20 minutes.

NUTRITION:

20 pieces, each with a trace of carbohydrates, a trace of fiber, and 4 grams of protein.

27. Cloud Eggs

Easy and yummy breakfast for a weekday that you can make in less than half an hour.

Serves: 2 servings

INGREDIENTS:

Nonstick cooking spray

One teaspoon Tuscan Fantasy Seasoning (or just about any other seasoning, SH, or otherwise!)

2 T grated parmesan cheese

Six whole eggs, whites, and yolks separated.

DIRECTIONS:

1. Preheat the oven to 450 ° C.

2. Line a silicone baking mat (or parchment paper) with a cookie sheet and lightly spray it with a nonstick cooking spray.

3. Put the egg whites and yolks apart. If you put each yolk in a separate jar, they can be "slipped" later into the clouds. You can put them in one bowl and then, in the next step, carefully spoon them out one by one.

4. Whip the whites into stiff peaks using an electric mixer, for around 3 minutes.

5. Fold the Parmesan cheese gently and use a spatula to season the egg whites.

6. Spoon the egg white mixture into six mounds onto the prepared baking sheet.

7. Gently indent the centers using the backside of a wide tablespoon to create nests for the egg yolks.

8. Remove the clouds from the oven and gently add the center of each puff with one yolk. Season to taste with salt and pepper, or better yet, give them a pinch of Seasoning Splash of Desperation to make them WOW.

9. Bake for about three more minutes, until the yolks are set. If needed, garnish it with fresh herbs.

10. Serve it warm.

28. Onion Eggs

This is not only a nice party snack but a nutritious breakfast too.

Preparation Time: 5 min

Cooking Time: 10 min

INGREDIENTS:

5 teaspoons very finely minced sweet red onion

A teaspoon of spicy brown or Dijon mustard 10 tablespoons of mayonnaise 12 hard-boiled eggs

6-8 drops Tabasco

2/4 teaspoon salt or Vega-Sal

DIRECTIONS:

1. Cut the eggs in two, and then separate the yolks gently in a mixing cup.

2. Mash the yolks using a fork. Combine the mustard, mayonnaise, Tabasco, onion, and salt and blend well until fluffy.

3. Put the egg yolk paste back into the hollows of egg white.

NUTRITION:

24 halves, each with a bit of carbohydrate, a fiber trace, and 5 grams of protein.

29. Hammond Eggs

Deviled ham provides these eggs with a kind of country blow.

Preparation Time: 5 min

Cooking Time: 10 min

INGREDIENTS:

Paprika

2/4 teaspoon of salt

6 tablespoons of mayonnaise

8 teaspoons of spicy brown mustard

1 can (5 ounces) of deviled ham

12 hard-boiled eggs

DIRECTIONS:

1. Split the eggs into two half's, then gently remove the yolks in a mixing cup.

2. Using a fork, mash the yolks. Add ham, mustard, mayonnaise, and salt and blend until fluffy.

3. Place the white egg paste back in the hollows. Dust a little paprika for spice.

NUTRITION:

Makes 24 halves, each with 2 grams of carbohydrates, a fiber trace, and 4-6 grams of protein.

30. Deviled Eggs

These are everyone's potluck personal favorite.

Preparation Time: 5 min

Cooking Time: 10 min

INGREDIENTS:

Paprika

12 hard-boiled eggs

10 tablespoons mayonnaise

4 teaspoons spicy brown or Dijon mustard 2/4 teaspoon salt or Vega-Sal

DIRECTIONS:

1. Split the eggs in half and carefully separate the yolks into a mixing bowl.

2. Mash the yolks using a fork. Add in the mustard, mayonnaise, and salt, and mix until fluffy.

3. Put the egg white paste back into the hollows. For flavor, sprinkle with a little paprika.

NUTRITION:

24 halves, each with a bit of carbohydrate, a fiber trace, and 3 grams of protein.

31. Cajun Eggs

For any event, these are some tasty treats.

Preparation Time: 5 min

Cooking Time: 10 min

INGREDIENTS:

6 hard-boiled eggs

1/3 cup mayonnaise

A teaspoons horseradish mustard

1 teaspoon Cajun Seasoning

DIRECTIONS:

1. Cut the eggs in two, and then separate the yolks gently in a mixing cup.

2. With a fork, mash the yolks. Whisk in the mayonnaise and mustard, and then blend until fluffy.

3. Adding the Cajun spice mix well.

4. Spoon the egg white paste back into the eggs.

NUTRITION:

24halves, each with 1 gram of carbohydrates, a fiber trace, and 3 grams of protein.

32. Fish Eggs

That is fish with eggs, not fish eggs. If you felt you couldn't go to an extravagant party with stuffed eggs, these should change your opinion.

Preparation Time: 5 min

Cooking Time: 10 min

INGREDIENTS:

1/4 teaspoon salt

tablespoon jarred, grated horseradish

1/2 cup moist smoked salmon, mashed fine

tablespoons sour cream

tablespoons mayonnaise

A teaspoon of finely minced sweet red onion

12 hard-boiled eggs

DIRECTIONS:

1. Cut the eggs in two, and then separate the yolks gently in a mixing cup.

2. With a fork, mash the yolks. Add the whipped cream, mayonnaise, tuna, onion, horseradish, salt, and blend until the mixture is smooth.

3. Spoon the egg white paste back into the eggs.

NUTRITION:

24 halves, each with a bit of carbohydrate, a bit of fiber, and 3 grams of protein.

33. Buttery Eggs

Curried, buttery, and perfect!

Preparation Time: 5 min

Cooking Time: 10 min

INGREDIENTS:

1 teaspoon salt

1/2 teaspoon Tabasco

2/3 cup mayonnaise

clove garlic, crushed

1 scallion, including the crisp part of the green shoot, finely minced

teaspoon curry powder

2 tablespoon butter

12 hard-boiled eggs

DIRECTIONS:

1. Cut the eggs in two, and then separate the yolks gently in a mixing cup.

2. Melt the butter in a tiny, heavy skillet over a low fire. Put in the garlic and curry powder, and mix for about 2 minutes.

3. Scrape the yolks into the butter mixture. Add in the mayonnaise, salt, scallion, and Tabasco, and blend until smooth.

4. Spoon the egg white paste back into the hollows.

NUTRITION:

24 halves, each with 1 gram of carbohydrates, a bit of fiber, and 3 grams of protein.

34. Parmesan Dip

Serve with pepper strips, cucumber circles, celery sticks, or low-carb fiber crackers with this party classic.

Preparation Time: 15 min

Cooking Time: 45 min

INGREDIENTS:

Paprika

teaspoons of jarred or 2 clove garlic, crushed, chopped garlic

cup grated Parmesan cheese

2 cup mayonnaise

2 can (26 ounces) artichoke hearts

DIRECTIONS:

1. Preheat your oven to 325 ° F.

2. Drain and cut the hearts of an artichoke.

3. Add the heart of the artichoke with the cheese, mayonnaise, and garlic and mix well.

4. In a tight, oven-proof casserole, place the mixture, sprinkle some paprika on top, and bake for 45 minutes.

NUTRITION:

4 servings, each with 3 grams of carbohydrates and a gram of fiber, for 2 grams of usable carbs and 10 grams of protein.

35. Easy Dip

This simple dip tastes yummy with all kinds of raw veggies; consider pairing it with peppers, celery, broccoli, cucumber, or whatever else you have on board.

Preparation Time: 5 min

Cooking Time: None

INGREDIENTS:

1 teaspoon salt or Vega-Sal

a heaping tablespoon of dry dill weed

1/2 small onion

2-pint sour cream

DIRECTIONS:

1. In a food processor, place the onion, sour cream, dill weed, and salt and grind before the onion disappears. (If you don't have a food processor, thinly dice the onion and only stir it all together.)

2. You can eat it straight away, but if you leave it to cool for a few hours, it tastes much better.

NUTRITION:

1 pint, containing 25 grams of carbohydrates and 1 gram of fiber, for a total of 24 grams of usable carbs and 16 grams of protein in the batch (This is easily enough for 12 to 20 people, so no one's going to get more than a few grams of carbs.)

36. Spinach Artichoke Dip

This is a slight, similarly tasty variation of a previous recipe. Just bear in mind that it requires twice as much dip.

Preparation Time: 15 min

Cooking Time: 1 hour

INGREDIENTS:

Paprika

4 cloves garlic, crushed, or 4 teaspoons jarred chopped garlic

4 cups grated Parmesan cheese

4 cups mayonnaise

package frozen chopped spinach (20 ounces), thawed

can (26 ounces) artichoke hearts

DIRECTIONS:

1. Drain and chop the hearts of an artichoke.

2. In a big casserole, mix the mayonnaise, spinach, cheese, and garlic (a 6-cup dish is just the best one). Sprinkle with minced paprika.

3. Bake for 50 to 60 minutes at 325 ° F.

NUTRITION:

8 servings, each with 4 grams of carbohydrates and 2 grams of fiber, for 2 grams of usable carbs and 10 grams of protein.

37. Clam Dip

This would make a decent lunch with some celery sticks and pepper strips for popping. Of course, with green pepper, celery, cucumber rounds, or fiber crackers for you, and chips or crackers for None-low-carvers, you should serve it at events too.

Preparation Time: 5 min

Cooking Time: None

INGREDIENTS:

Salt or Vega-Sal

4 cans (12 ounces each) minced clams, drained

10 to 12 scallions, including the crisp part of the green shoot, minced

tablespoon Dijon mustard

to 4 teaspoons Worcestershire sauce

1 cup mayonnaise

packages (16 ounces each) cream cheese, softened

Pepper

DIRECTIONS:

Combine well with all the items, and cool. To do this, a food processor or blender serves well, or you might use an electric mixer if you want to keep bits of clam.

NUTRITION:

12 servings, each with just under 4 grams of carbohydrates, a bit of fiber, and 10 grams of protein.

Chapter IX: Lean and green recipes

Today we are talking about lean, fast, and delicious recipes perfect to offer to your loved ones. Even if you are on a diet, you must not give up on taste and imagination.

Dieting doesn't necessarily mean eating sad and bland dishes! However, with my ideas, you can organize a light dinner with the family... without saying anything! The recipes will be so tasty that no one will wonder if they are dietary or not!

38. Shrimp & Zucchini

Serving: 2

Prep time: 10 min

Cooking time: 30 min

INGREDIENTS:

1 lb shrimp, peeled and deveined

1 zucchini, chopped

1 summer squash, chopped

2 tbsp olive oil

1/2 small onion, chopped

1/2 tsp paprika

1/2 tsp garlic powder

1/2 tsp onion powder

Pepper

Salt

DIRECTIONS:

In a bowl, mix together paprika, garlic powder, onion powder, pepper, and salt. Add shrimp and toss well.

Heat 1 tablespoon of oil in a pan over medium heat.

Add shrimp and cook for 2 minutes on each side or until shrimp turns pink.

Transfer shrimp on a plate.

Add remaining oil to a pan.

Add onion, summer squash, and zucchini and cook for 6-8 minutes or until vegetables are softened.

Return shrimp to the pan and cook for 1 minute.

NUTRITION:

Calories 215, Fat 4, Carbs 15, Protein 6, Sodium 422

39. Baked Dijon Salmon

Serving: 2

Prep time: 10 min

Cooking time: 30 min

INGREDIENTS:

1 1/2 lbs salmon

1/4 cup Dijon mustard

1/4 cup fresh parsley, chopped

1 tbsp garlic, chopped

1 tbsp olive oil

1 tbsp fresh lemon juice

Pepper

Salt

DIRECTIONS:

Preheat the oven to 375 F. Line baking sheet with parchment paper.

Arrange salmon fillets on a prepared baking sheet.

In a small bowl, mix together garlic, oil, lemon juice, Dijon mustard, parsley, pepper, and salt.

Brush salmon top with garlic mixture.

Bake for 18-20 minutes.

Serve and enjoy.

NUTRITION:

Calories 254, Fat 6, Carbs 8, Protein 21, Sodium 338

40. Optavia Tomato Basil Soup

Serving: 2

Prep time: 10 min

Cooking time: 10 min

INGREDIENTS:

1 cup tomatoes, chopped

½ cup of water

1 cup basil leaves

1 tablespoon low-sodium and low-fat cheese, shredded

DIRECTIONS:

Place the tomatoes in a saucepan. Pour water. Close the lid.

Turn the heat to medium and allow the tomatoes to boil.

Using a handheld blender, puree the tomatoes while still in a pan.

Add in the basil leaves and allow to cook for another 2 minutes.

Scoop in bowls and serve with ½ tablespoon each shredded cheese.

NUTRITION:

Calories 137, Fat 2, Carbs 18, Protein 6, Sodium 515

41. Cauliflower with Kale Pesto

Serving: 2

Prep time: 5 min

Cooking time: 2 min

INGREDIENTS:

3 cups cauliflower, cut into florets

3 cups raw kale, stems removed

2 cups fresh basil

2 tablespoons extra virgin olive oil

3 tablespoons lemon juice

3 cloves of garlic

¼ teaspoon salt

DIRECTIONS:

Put enough water in a pot and bring to a boil over medium flame. Blanch the cauliflower for 2 minutes. Drain, then place in a bowl of ice-cold water for 5 minutes. Drain again.

In a blender, add the rest of the ingredients. Pulse until smooth.

Pour the pesto over the cooked cauliflower.

NUTRITION:

Calories 146, Fat 2, Carbs 12, Protein 6, Sodium 390

41. Lean and Green Cauliflower Salad

Serving: 2

Prep time: 10 min

Cooking time: 3 min

INGREDIENTS:

1 cup cauliflower florets

¼ cup apple cider vinegar

1 tablespoon Tuscan seasoning

DIRECTIONS:

Add all ingredients into a bowl and toss to combine.

Allow resting in the fridge for at least 30 minutes before serving.

NUTRITION:

Calories 48, Fat 1, Carbs 10, Protein 4, Sodium 580

43. Lean and Green Garlic Chicken with Zoodles

Serving: 2

Prep time: 10 min

Cooking time: 10 min

INGREDIENTS:

1 ½ pound boneless and skinless chicken breasts, cut into bite-sized pieces

6 slices sun-dried tomatoes

1 teaspoon chopped garlic

1 cup low-fat plain Greek yogurt

½ cup chicken broth, low sodium

½ teaspoon garlic powder

½ teaspoon Italian seasoning

1 cup spinach, chopped

1 ½ cup zucchini, cut into thin noodles

DIRECTIONS:

Place 2 tablespoons water in a pan and heat over low-medium flame. Water sauté the chicken for 3 minutes while constantly stirring until the sides are slightly golden.

Stir in the tomatoes and garlic and stir for another 3 minutes. Add in the yogurt, chicken broth, garlic powder, and Italian seasoning. Cover with lid and allow to simmer for at least 7 minutes.

Stir in the spinach last. Cook for another 2 minutes.

Place the zucchini noodles in a deep dish and pour over the chicken. Toss the noodles to coat with the sauce.

Serve immediately.

NUTRITION:

Calories 270, Fat 4, Carbs 16, Protein 6, Sodium 521

43. Lean and Green "Macaroni"

Serving: 2

Prep time: 10 min

Cooking time: 30 min

INGREDIENTS:

2 tablespoons yellow onion, diced

5 ounces 95-97% lean ground beef

2 tablespoons light thousand island dressing 1/8 teaspoon apple cider vinegar 1/8 teaspoon onion powder

3 cups Romaine lettuce, shredded

2 tablespoons low-fat cheddar cheese, shredded

1-ounce dill pickle slices

1 teaspoon sesame seeds

DIRECTIONS:

Put 3 tablespoons of water in a pan and heat over a medium-low flame. Water sauté the onions for 30 seconds before adding the beef. Sauté the beef for 4 minutes while stirring constantly.

Add in the thousand island dressing, apple cider vinegar, and onion powder. Close the lid and keep on cooking for 5 minutes. Remove the lid and allow it to simmer until the sauce thickens. Turn off the heat and allow the beef to rest and cool.

In a bowl, place the lettuce at the bottom and pour in the beef. Layer with cheddar cheese and pickles. Sprinkle with sesame on top.

NUTRITION:

Calories 412, Fat 8, Carbs 18, Protein 4, Sodium 643

44. Lean and Green Broccoli Taco

Serving: 2

Prep time: 10 min

Cooking time: 15 min

INGREDIENTS:

4 ounces 95-97% lean ground beef

¼ cup Roma tomatoes, chopped

¼ teaspoon garlic powder

¼ teaspoon onion powder

1 ¼ cup broccoli, cut into bite-sized pieces

A pinch of red pepper flakes

1-ounce low-sodium cheddar cheese, shredded

DIRECTIONS:

Place 3 tablespoons of water in a pan and heat over medium flame. Water sauté the beef and tomatoes for 5 minutes until the tomatoes are wilted. Add in the garlic and onion powder and stir for another 3 minutes.

Add the broccoli and close the lid. Cook for another 5 minutes.

Garnish with red pepper flakes and cheddar cheese on top.

NUTRITION:

Calories 412, Fat 6, Carbs 20, Protein 6, Sodium 421

45. Lean and Green Crunchy Chicken Tacos

Serving: 2

Prep time: 10 min

Cooking time: 10 min

INGREDIENTS:

½ cup low sodium chicken stock

2 chicken breasts, minced

1 red onion, chopped

1 clove of garlic, minced

3 plum tomatoes, chopped

1 teaspoon cumin powder

1 teaspoon cinnamon powder

1 teaspoon ground coriander

1 red onion, chopped

½ red chili, chopped

1 tablespoon lime juice

Meat from 1 ripe avocado

1 cucumber, sliced into thick rounds

DIRECTIONS:

Place a tablespoon of chicken stock in a pan and heat over medium flame. Water sauté the chicken, onion, garlic, and tomatoes for 4 minutes or until the tomatoes have wilted.

Season with cumin, cinnamon, and coriander. Reduce the heat to low and cook for another 5 minutes. Set aside and allow to cool.

In a bowl, mix together the onion, chili, lime juice, and mashed avocado.

This is salsa.

Scoop the salsa and top on sliced cucumber. Top with cooked chicken.

NUTRITION:

Calories 447, Fat 8, Carbs 12, Protein 24, Sodium 321

46. Optavia-Approved Vegetarian Zucchini Lasagna

Serving: 2

Prep time: 10 min

Cooking time: 10 min

INGREDIENTS:

1 ¼ pounds zucchini, sliced into lasagna

¼ cup chopped fresh spinach

1 ½ cup sugar-free and low-sodium marinara sauce 2/3 cup mozzarella cheese, shredded

1 cup part-skim ricotta cheese

Fresh basil for garnish

DIRECTIONS:

Preheat the oven to 3750F for 5 minutes.

Place the zucchini slices in a dish and layer with spinach, marinara sauce, mozzarella, and ricotta cheese. Repeat the process until several layers are formed.

Top with basil.

Place in the oven and bake for 10 minutes.

NUTRITION:

Calories 412, Fat 9, Carbs 16, Protein 6, Sodium 890

47. Lean and Green Chicken Chili

Serving: 2

Prep time: 10 min

Cooking time: 45 min

INGREDIENTS:

1-pound boneless skinless chicken breast, chopped

1 teaspoon ground cumin

1 cup chopped poblano pepper

½ cup chopped onion

1 clove of garlic, minced

2 cups low-sodium chicken broth

1 cup rehydrated pinto beans

1 cup chopped tomatoes

2 tablespoons minced cilantro

DIRECTIONS:

Place all ingredients except the cilantro in a pressure cooker.

Close the lid and set the vent to the sealing position.

Cook on high for 45 minutes until the beans are soft.

Garnish with cilantro before serving.

NUTRITION:

Calories 229, Fat 12, Carbs 23, Protein 21, Sodium 421

48. Avocado, Citrus, And Shrimp Salad

Serving: 2

Prep time: 10 min

Cooking time: 4 min

INGREDIENTS:

1 head green leaf lettuce

1 avocado

½ pound wild-caught shrimp

2 tablespoons olive oil

Juice of 1 lemon

DIRECTIONS:

Place the lettuce in a bowl and top with mashed avocado meat.

Clean the shrimps by deveining and removing the head.

Heat oil in a skillet over medium-low heat and heat the oil. Cook the shrimps for 2 minutes on each side.

Place the shrimps on top of mashed avocado and drizzle with lemon juice.

NUTRITION:

Calories 359, Fat 5, Carbs 16, Protein 6, Sodium 585

49. Lean and Green Broccoli Alfredo

Serving: 2

Prep time: 10 min

Cooking time: 2 min

INGREDIENTS:

2 heads of broccoli, cut into florets

2 tablespoons lemon juice, freshly squeezed

½ cup cashew, soaked for 2 hours in water then drained 2 tablespoons white miso, low sodium 2 teaspoons Dijon mustard

Freshly cracked black pepper

DIRECTIONS:

Boil water in a pot over medium flame. Blanch the broccoli for 2 minutes, then place it in a bowl of iced water. Drain.

In a food processor, place the remaining ingredients and pulse until smooth.

Pour the alfredo sauce over the broccoli. Toss to coat with the sauce.

NUTRITION:

Calories 156, Fat 4, Carbs 21, Protein 4, Sodium 219

50. Lean and Green Steak Machine

Serving: 2

Prep time: 10 min

Cooking time: 10 min

INGREDIENTS:

1/2 teaspoon extra virgin olive oil

2 ounces Sirloin steak, 98% lean

Salt and pepper to taste

1 zucchini, cut into long thin strips

1 onion, chopped

6 ounces asparagus, blanched

4 ounces peas, blanched

DIRECTIONS:

Heat olive oil in a skillet. Season the steak with salt and pepper to taste.

Place in the skillet and sear the steak for 5 minutes on each side. Allow resting for five minutes before slicing into strips.

Place the remaining ingredients in a bowl and season with salt and pepper to taste

Top with steak strips, then toss to combine all ingredients.

NUTRITION:

Calories 174, Fat 8, Carbs 23, Protein 8, Sodium 20

51. Garlic Shrimp Zucchini Noodles

Serving: 2

Prep time: 10 min

Cooking time: 4 min

INGREDIENTS:

16 ounces uncooked shrimps, shelled and deveined

1 tablespoon olive oil

1 cup cherry tomatoes, cut in half

8 cups zucchini strips

2 tablespoons minced garlic

1 teaspoon dried oregano

½ teaspoon chili powder

½ teaspoon salt

DIRECTIONS:

Brush the shrimps with olive oil. Place on a skillet and cook for 2 minutes on all sides or until pink. Set aside.

Place the rest of the ingredients in a bowl and add the shrimps. Season with salt, then toss to coat the ingredients.

NUTRITION:

Calories 633, Fat 6, Carbs 32, Protein 12, Sodium 509

52. Broccoli Kale Salmon Burgers

Serving: 2

Prep time: 10 min

Cooking time: 30 min

INGREDIENTS:

2 eggs

½ cup onion, chopped

½ cup broccoli, chopped

½ cup kale, chopped

½ tsp garlic powder

2 tbsp lemon juice

½ cup almond flour

15 oz can salmon, drained and bones removed ½ tsp salt

DIRECTIONS:

Line one plate with parchment paper and set aside.

Add all ingredients into the large bowl and mix until well combined.

Make five equal shapes of patties from the mixture and place them on a prepared plate.

Place the plate in the refrigerator for 30 minutes.

Spray a large pan with cooking spray and heat over medium heat.

Once the pan is hot, add patties and cook for 5-7 minutes per side.

Serve and enjoy.

NUTRITION:

Calories 221, Fat 6, Carbs 18, Protein 8, Sodium 321

53. Pan-Seared Cod

Serving: 2

Prep time: 10 min

Cooking time: 25 min

INGREDIENTS:

1 ¾ lbs cod fillets

1 tbsp ranch seasoning

4 tsp olive oil

DIRECTIONS:

Heat oil in a large pan over medium-high heat.

Season fish fillets with ranch seasoning.

Once the oil is hot, place fish fillets in a pan and cook for 6-8 minutes on each side.

Serve immediately and enjoy it.

NUTRITION:

Calories 204, Fat 6, Carbs 12, Protein 6, Sodium 643

54. Quick Lemon Pepper Salmon

Serving: 2

Prep time: 10 min

Cooking time: 18 min

INGREDIENTS:

1 ½ lbs salmon fillets

½ tsp ground black pepper

1 tsp dried oregano

2 garlic cloves, minced

¼ cup olive oil

1 lemon juice

1 tsp sea salt

DIRECTIONS:

In a large bowl, mix together lemon juice, olive oil, garlic, oregano, black pepper, and salt.

Add fish fillets in bowl and coat well with the marinade, and place in the refrigerator for 15 minutes.

Preheat the grill.

Brush grill grates with oil.

Place marinated salmon fillets on a hot grill and cook for 4 minutes, then turn salmon fillets to the other side and cook for 4 minutes more.

NUTRITION:

Calories 340, Fat 6, Carbs 31, Protein 28, Sodium 321

55. Healthy Salmon Salad

Serving: 2

Prep time: 10 min

Cooking time: 20 min

INGREDIENTS:

2 salmon fillets

2 tbsp olive oil

¼ cup onion, chopped

1 cucumber, peeled and sliced

1 avocado, diced

2 tomatoes, chopped

4 cups baby spinach

Pepper

Salt

DIRECTIONS:

Heat oil in a pan over medium-high heat.

Season salmon fillets with pepper and salt. Place fish fillets in a pan and cook for 4-5 minutes.

Turn fish fillets and cook for 2-3 minutes more.

Divide remaining ingredients evenly between two bowls, then top with cooked fish fillet.

NUTRITION:

Calories 320, Fat 8, Carbs 21, Protein 8, Sodium 650

56. Pan-Seared Tilapia

Serving: 2

Prep time: 10 min

Cooking time: 18 min

INGREDIENTS:

18 oz tilapia fillets

¼ tsp lemon pepper

½ tsp parsley flakes

¼ tsp garlic powder

1 tsp Cajun seasoning

½ tsp dried oregano

2 tbsp olive oil

DIRECTIONS:

Heat olive oil in a pan over medium heat.

Season fish fillets with lemon pepper, parsley flakes, garlic powder, Cajun seasoning, and oregano.

Place fish fillets in the pan and cook for 3-4 minutes on each side.

NUTRITION:

Calories 321, Fat 5, Carbs 22, Protein 21, Sodium 387

57. Creamy Broccoli Soup

Serving: 2

Prep time: 10 min

Cooking time: 35 min

INGREDIENTS:

20 oz frozen broccoli, thawed and chopped ¼ tsp nutmeg

4 cups vegetable broth

1 potato, peeled and chopped

2 garlic cloves, peeled and chopped

1 large onion, chopped

1 tbsp olive oil

Pepper

Salt

DIRECTIONS:

Heat oil in a large saucepan over medium heat.

Add garlic and onion and sauté until onion is tender.

Add potato, broccoli, and broth and bring to boil. Turn heat to low and simmer for 15 minutes or until vegetables are tender.

Using a blender, puree the soup until smooth. Season soup with nutmeg, pepper, and salt.

NUTRITION:

Calories 184, Fat 6, Carbs 18, Protein 21, Sodium 342

58. Tuna Muffins

Serving: 2

Prep time: 10 min

Cooking time: 35 min

INGREDIENTS:

2 eggs, lightly beaten

1 can tuna, flaked

1 tsp cayenne pepper

1/4 cup mayonnaise

1 celery stalk, chopped

1 1/2 cups cheddar cheese, shredded

1/4 cup sour cream

Pepper

Salt

DIRECTIONS:

Preheat the oven to 350 F. Grease muffin tin and set aside.

Add all ingredients into the large bowl and mix until well combined and pour into the prepared muffin tin.

Bake for 25 minutes.

NUTRITION:

Calories 434, Fat 6, Carbs 28, Protein 4, Sodium 548

Chapter X: Meat and fish dishes

From burgers in the company to breaded meatballs, from baked salmon fillet to octopus salad: meat and fish are the protagonists of the Italian culinary tradition. This section will find the most popular recipes, ideal for both Sunday lunch and dinner on the fly. A nice grilled steak or a pan-fried scallop, perhaps together with tasty sauces? You just have to choose; in any case, you will bring a masterpiece to the table, still eating in a healthy and lean way.

59. Asparagus and Crabmeat Frittata

Preparation Time: 10–15 minutes

Cooking Time: 15–20 minutes

Servings: 1

INGREDIENTS:

1½ tablespoon extra-virgin olive oil

1 pound asparagus

1/2 teaspoon salt

1 ½ teaspoon black pepper

1/2 teaspoon sweet paprika

1/2 pound lump crabmeat

1/2 tablespoon finely cut chives

¼ cup basil chopped

1/2 cups liquid egg substitute

DIRECTIONS:

1. Deter the tough ends of the asparagus and cut it into bite-sized pieces.

2. Preheat an oven to 375°F.

3. In a 12-Inch to a 14-inch oven-proof, non-stick skillet, warm the olive oil and sweat the asparagus until tender—season with pepper, paprika, and salt.

4. In a mixing bowl, add the chives, crabmeat, and basil.

5. Pour in the liquid egg substitute and mix until combined.

6. With the cooked asparagus, pour the crab and egg mixture into the skillet, then stir to combine. Bake over low to medium heat until the eggs start bubbling.

7. Place the skillet inside the oven. Then, bake for about 15–20 minutes. Wait until the eggs are golden brown. Serve the dish warm.

NUTRITION:

Calories: 340

Protein: 50g

Carbohydrates: 14g

Fats: 10g

60. Grilled Chicken Power Bowl with Green Goddess Dressing

Preparation Time: 30 minutes

Cooking Time: 15 minutes

Servings: 1

INGREDIENTS:

1/3 boneless, skinless chicken breasts

1/8 teaspoon each salt & pepper

1/4 cup rice or cubed kabocha squash

1/4 cup diced zucchini

1/4 cup rice yellow summer squash

1/4 cup rice broccoli

2 cherry tomatoes halved

1 radish, sliced thin

1/4 cup shredded red cabbage

1/8 cup hemp or pumpkin seeds

Green goddess dressing

½ cup low-fat plain Greek yogurt

1/4 cup fresh basil

1/4 clove garlic

1 tablespoon lemon juice

¼ teaspoon each salt & pepper

DIRECTIONS:

1. Preheat oven to 350°F.

2. Season chicken with salt and pepper.

3. Roast chicken for about 10–12 minutes or until it reaches a temperature of 165°F. When done, dismiss from oven and set aside to rest about 5 minutes. Cut into bite-sized pieces and keep warm.

4. While the chicken rests, steam riced kabocha squash, yellow summer squash, zucchini, and broccoli in a covered microwave-proof bowl for about 5 minutes till tender.

5. For the dressing, arrange the ingredients in a blender and puree till smooth.

6. To serve into four individual serving bowls, put an equal amount of the riced veggie mixture. Make sure to add an equal amount of cherry tomatoes, radishes, and shredded cabbage to each bowl. Each bowl should also contain a quarter of the chicken and one tablespoon of seeds—drizzle dressing on top. Enjoy!

NUTRITION:

Calories: 300

Protein: 43g

Carbohydrates: 12g

Fats: 10g

61. Bacon Cheeseburger

Preparation Time: 5 minutes

Cooking Time: 15 minutes

Servings: 1

INGREDIENTS:

1/4 pound lean ground beef

¼ cup chopped yellow onion

1/4 clove garlic, minced

1/4 tablespoon yellow mustard

1/4 tablespoon Worcestershire sauce

1/8 teaspoon salt

Cooking spray

1 ultra-thin slice cheddar cheese, cut into six equal-sized rectangular pieces

1piece of turkey bacon, each cut into eight evenly sized rectangular pieces

3 dill pickle chips

1–2 green leaf lettuce leaves, torn into 24 small square-shaped pieces

2 cherry tomatoes, sliced in half

DIRECTIONS:

1. Preheat oven to 400°F.

2. Combine the garlic, salt, onion, Worcestershire sauce, and beef in a medium-sized bowl, and mix well.

3. Form mixture into 24 small meatballs. Put meatballs onto a foil-lined baking sheet and cook for 12–15 minutes. Leave oven.

4. Top every meatball with a piece of cheese, then go back to the oven till cheese melts, about 2 to 3 minutes. Let meatballs cool.

5. To assemble bites: on a toothpick layer, a cheese-covered meatball, piece of bacon, piece of lettuce, pickle chip, and a tomato half.

NUTRITION:

Calories: 303

Protein: 15g

Carbohydrates: 30g

Fats: 14g

62. Ancho Tilapia on Cauliflower Rice

Preparation Time: 10 minutes

Cooking Time: 20 minutes

Servings: 1

INGREDIENTS:

1/2 lbs. tilapia

1/4 teaspoon lime juice

1/4 teaspoon salt

1/4 tablespoon ground ancho pepper

1/4 teaspoon ground cumin

3/4 tablespoon extra-virgin olive oil

1/16 cup toasted pumpkin seeds

3/2 cups cauliflower rice minutes

1/4 cup coarsely chopped fresh coriander

DIRECTIONS:

1. Preheat oven to 450°F.

2. Dress tilapia with lime juice and set aside.

3. Combine cumin, ancho pepper, and salt in a bowl—season tilapia with spice mixture.

4. Lay tilapia on a baking sheet or casserole dish and bake for 7 minutes.

5. In the meantime, in a big skillet, sweat the cauliflower rice in olive oil till tender, about 2–3 minutes.

6. Blend the pumpkin seeds and coriander into the rice. Dismiss from heat and serve.

NUTRITION:

Calories: 350

Protein: 51g

Carbohydrates: 10g

Fats: 10g

63. Turkey Caprese Meatloaf Cups

Preparation Time: 10 minutes

Cooking Time: 35 minutes

Servings: 1

INGREDIENTS:

1/4 large egg

1/4 pounds ground turkey breast

1 piece of sun-dried tomatoes, drained and chopped

¼ cup fresh basil leaves, chopped

1-oz. low-fat fresh mozzarella, shredded

½ teaspoon garlic powder

¼ teaspoon salt and ½ teaspoon pepper, to taste

DIRECTIONS:

1. Preheat oven to 400°F.

2. Beat the egg in a big mixing bowl.

3. Add the remaining ingredients and mix everything with your hands until evenly combined.

4. Spray a 12-cup muffin tin and divide the turkey mixture among the muffin cups, pressing the mix. Cook in the preheated oven till the turkey is well-cooked for about 25–30 minutes.

5. Chill the meatloaves entirely and store them in a container in the fridge for up to 5 days.

NUTRITION:

Calories: 149

Protein: 17g

Carbohydrates: 4.5g

Fats: 6g

64. Chicken Lo Mein

Preparation Time: 15 minutes

Cooking Time: 15 minutes

Servings: 1

INGREDIENTS:

1/2 tablespoon + 1/2 teaspoon sesame oil, divided

220g boneless. skinless chicken breasts, sliced ¼ teaspoon ground black pepper

1/4 tablespoon soy sauce

1/4 tablespoon oyster sauce

1/4 garlic clove, minced

1/2 teaspoon fresh ginger root

1/2 spring onions, trimmed and sliced with white and green parts separated

25g fresh mushrooms, divided

1/4 medium red bell pepper, membranes, and seeds removed
1/2 medium zucchinis (400g), cut, sliced

DIRECTIONS:

1. In a skillet, heat one-teaspoon sesame oil over medium-high heat. Put the shredded chicken, season with black pepper, and cook until chicken is done (internal temperature about 165°F). Dismiss from wok or skillet and set aside.

2. While the chicken cooks, prepare the sauce by combining the oyster sauce, soy sauce, and two tablespoons sesame oil in a bowl and whisking together. Set aside.

3. With the same skillet used to cook the chicken, heat one teaspoon sesame oil and put the garlic, ginger, and white spring onion pieces; cook until fragrant, about 1 minute. Put the mushrooms and bell peppers and continue to cook until just tender, about 3 minutes. Add zucchini noodles and toss to combine.

4. Pour in the sauce and put the chicken; cook until zucchini is tender, and the mixture should be heated by about 3 to 5 minutes.

5. Garnish with green parts of spring onions.

NUTRITION:

Calories: 330

Protein: 48g

Carbohydrates: 9g

Fats: 10g

65. Sheet Pan Chicken Fajita Lettuce Wraps

Preparation Time: 10 minutes

Cooking Time: 30 minutes

Servings: 1

INGREDIENTS:

1/2 b. chicken breast, thinly sliced into strips

1/2 bell peppers, thinly sliced into strips 1/2 teaspoon olive oil

1/2 teaspoon fajita seasoning

Juice of half a lime

1 leaf from a romaine heart

Optional ¼ cup plain non-fat Greek yogurt

DIRECTIONS:

1. Preheat oven to about 400 °F.

2. Merge every ingredient except for lettuce in a big, re-sealable plastic bag. Stir well; make sure to coat chicken and vegetables with oil and seasoning equally.

3. Release contents of the bag equally on a foil-lined baking sheet. Cook for 30 minutes until the chicken is well cooked.

4. Serve on lettuce leaves, topped with Greek yogurt.

NUTRITION:

Calories: 352

Protein: 20g

Carbohydrates: 4.1g

Fats: 12g

66. Cauliflower Pizza with Chicken and Tzatziki

Preparation Time: 10 minutes

Cooking Time: 60 minutes

Servings: 1

INGREDIENTS:

1 cup rice cauliflower

1/2 egg

1/2 tablespoon low-fat parmesan cheese

¼ teaspoon salt, divided

1/4 pound boneless, skinless chicken breast, cut into fine strips

2 kalamata olives, pitted and chopped

½ teaspoon Italian seasoning

¼ teaspoon ground black pepper

1/4 cup reduced-fat, shredded mozzarella

½ cup peeled, seeded, and grated cucumber ½ cup low-fat plain Greek yogurt

½ teaspoon crushed garlic

DIRECTIONS:

1. Shed the cauliflower "rice" on a baking tin lined with parchment paper and cook at 425 °F for about 30 minutes.

2. Dismiss from the oven and allow it to cool.

3. In a paper towel, crush the cauliflower to remove any excess moisture.

4. In a big bowl, combine cauliflower with the parmesan cheese, eggs, and a quarter teaspoon salt. Stir to make a cohesive mix.

5. Put the cauliflower mixture onto the parchment-lined baking tin and press into a 12-inch circle shaped like a pizza.

6. Add the chicken strips, pepper, Italian seasoning, olives, and toss to combine.

7. Place chicken strips and olives on top of the cauliflower crust and spread with mozzarella cheese. Cook at about 430 °F for 20–25 minutes.

8. While the pizza bakes, make the tzatziki sauce. Combine the grated cucumbers, garlic, yogurt, and a quarter teaspoon of salt.

9. Slice the cauliflower pizza into four wedges and top each wedge with tzatziki.

NUTRITION:

Calories: 310

Protein: 50g

Carbohydrates: 11g

Fats: 12g

67. Chicken Chili

Preparation Time: 10 minutes

Cooking Time: 30 minutes

Servings: 1

INGREDIENTS:

1(¼ pound) boneless chicken breast, cut into bite-size pieces

1/4 tablespoon olive oil

1/4 cup green spring onion, diced

1/3 cup bell pepper, seeded and chopped

½ cup jalapenos, seeded and diced

½ cloves garlic, minced

½ teaspoon salt

1/4 teaspoon ground cumin

1/4 teaspoon coriander

1 cup chicken broth

1/2 cup water

½(7-oz.) cans green chilies

1 tablespoon thick canned coconut milk, chopped green onions, and coriander for garnish

DIRECTIONS:

1. Mince the chicken and veggies. Then place a big pot over medium-high heat. Put the peppers, oil, onions, jalapeno, and garlic up.

2. Sauté for 5 minutes, then put the chicken, spices, and salt. Sauté additional 5–8 minutes until chicken is cooked well. Place the green chilies, broth, and coconut milk.

3. Bring to the boil. Cook for 15–20 minutes and shred chicken. Serve topped with green onions and coriander.

NUTRITION:

Calories: 226

Protein: 20g

Carbohydrates: 19g

Fats: 8g

68. Eggplant Parmesan with Chops

Preparation Time: 5 minutes

Cooking Time: 40 minutes

Servings: 1

INGREDIENTS:

Bell peppers any color

Mushrooms

Vegetable broth

Cooking spray

Pepper

Salt

1/2 packet optavia pancake mix

1/3 large eggplant

Parmesan cheese

Pork chops

DIRECTIONS:

1. Using a non-stick pan, fry the pork chops. You should be using the cooking spray, then spray for 7 minutes on each side.

2. You also need to spray the glass cooking pan and lay chops on the bottom.

3. Followed by bell peppers around chops.

4. Put the mushrooms around chops

5. Next, place vegetable broth over chops filling the pan 1/4 inch from the bottom.

6. Put it in the oven and bake at 350 degrees for 30 minutes.

7. Make sure to peel the eggplant and slice.

8. Mix pancake batter as directed and add 1/8 teaspoon baking powder and two egg whites.

9. Then, mix and dip eggplant in batter fry until golden brown, set aside.

10. Remove chops from the oven, let cool.

11. Arrange 1/2 cup eggplant and 5-oz. peppers on a plate, scoop 1/4 cup marinara on top of the pork chop.

12. Top with 1/4 cup parmesan cheese.

13. Enjoy! It makes three green servings and one lean serving. Mushroom is an extra 1/2 cup; otherwise, just use it for flavor—put in the microwave for 30 seconds, serve hot.

NUTRITION:

Calories: 250

Carbohydrates: 14.5g

Fats: 15.9g

Protein: 25g

69. Spicy Tilapia with Spinach

Preparation Time: 10 minutes

Cooking Time: 30 minutes

Servings: 1

INGREDIENTS:

3 cups (1 small bunch) fresh spinach

9 oz. raw tilapia (should yield one (7 oz) cooked serving)

2 teaspoon olive oil or canola oil

1 cup or 2 small (2–2/5") canned tomatoes, make sure to chopped (to lessen the sodium content, you should make use of "no salt" canned tomatoes or fresh tomatoes)

¾ teaspoon paprika

¼ teaspoon red pepper flakes

¼ teaspoon garlic powder

½ teaspoon hot sauce

DIRECTIONS:

1. Begin by preheating the oven to 350 or 380° F.

2. Then paprika, red pepper flakes, garlic powder, and hot sauce.

3. Brush olive oil all over the fish.

4. Use seasoning mixture to coat the fish. Then place the tilapia flat in a baking pan.

5. Drain juice from canned tomatoes, place tomatoes on top of tilapia.

6. You need to cut the spinach into bite-sized pieces, place around tilapia in the pan.

7. Bake 30 minutes or until tilapia can be easily flaked with a fork and is opaque.

NUTRITION:

Calories: 350

Protein: 51g

Carbohydrates: 10g

Fats: 10g

70. Teriyaki Halibut

Preparation Time: 5 minutes

Cooking Time: 10 minutes

Servings: 1

INGREDIENTS:

2–1/4 cups cabbage, chopped

1 cup (1 small) zucchini, chopped

1 teaspoon Olive oil

(7 oz.) raw halibut (should yield one 6-oz cooked serving)

2 tablespoon teriyaki sauce

1/2 teaspoon cayenne pepper

Dash of salt and pepper (optional)

DIRECTIONS:

1. Start with sprinkling halibut with cayenne pepper or paprika and baste with teriyaki sauce. Next will be broiling it on tin foil 4" under a preheated broiler for 7 minutes.

2. Next, we will remove it in the oven and wrap in tin foil until ready to serve (this will continue to cook halibut).

3. Vegetables: Chop up zucchini and cabbage. Sauté olive oil, zucchini, and cabbage in a pan until slightly brown.

4. If desired, season it with salt and pepper to taste. Place on a plate and serve halibut on top of vegetables.

NUTRITION:

Calories: 510

Protein: 42.7g

Carbohydrates: 56.7g

Fats: 12.2g

71. Spiced Crockpot Roast Beef

Preparation Time: 20 minutes

Cooking Time: 4–8 hours

Servings: 1

INGREDIENTS:

1 tablespoon water

1/2 tablespoon black pepper

1/2 pounds raw, boneless beef chuck clod roast (this should result in six 5-oz cooked servings)

1/4 tablespoon soy sauce

1 teaspoon balsamic vinegar

1/2 teaspoon Worcestershire sauce

1/2 teaspoon dry mustard

½ teaspoon salt or salt substitute

1/2 cloves garlic, minced

1/2 cups celery, roughly diced

3/4 cups green beans, trimmed

1/6 cups whole mushrooms, trimmed

2 cups scallions, roughly chopped

DIRECTIONS:

1. Trim all visible fat from roast. Then rub black pepper and garlic onto roast.
2. Then produce several small shallow slits on top of the roast. Combine remaining spice blend ingredients in a bowl; pour over meat.
3. Then let it cook on low 8–10 hours or high 4–5 hours.
4. Lastly, add vegetables during the last 30–60 minutes of roasting.

NUTRITION:

Calories: 180

Protein: 24.7g

Carbohydrates: 14g

Fats: 5g

72. Spicy Garlic Lime Shrimp

Preparation Time: 10 minutes

Cooking Time: 15 minutes

Servings: 1

INGREDIENTS:

1 small 2–½" x 2" chopped green peppers

½ tablespoon lime juice

1/¾ pound (28 oz.) large, peeled, and deveined raw shrimp, peeled, and deveined; if using frozen, if you choose to use fully cooked shrimp, you need to use 1–1/3 lbs. (about 21 oz.) (both portions should yield three (7 oz) servings)

1 cup (2 small 2–2/5") fresh or canned tomatoes, diced (if using canned tomatoes, drain liquid)

½ tablespoon olive oil

8 oz. packages of hair noodles

½ clove garlic, pressed

SEASONING BLEND:

¼ teaspoon salt or salt substitute

¼ teaspoon ground black pepper

¼ teaspoon cayenne pepper

¼ teaspoon dried parsley flakes

¼ teaspoon garlic powder

¼ teaspoon paprika

1/8 teaspoon dried thyme

1/8 teaspoon onion powder

DIRECTIONS:

1. When you are using frozen shrimp, thaw. Also, devein and peel shrimp.

2. To make the seasoning blend, combine all the spices.

3. Drain liquid from noodles and rinse thoroughly, set aside.

4. Next is preheating a large skillet over medium heat. Once the pan is heated, add olive oil, and stir in pressed garlic cup. Immediately add shrimp, green bell peppers, and lime juice.

5. Make sure to sprinkle the entire seasoning blend over shrimp and peppers. Stir. Sauté shrimp and peppers 3–6 minutes.

6. They were followed by adding the drained noodles. You may continue to cook shrimp, peppers, and noodles. Wait for an additional 2–4 minutes or until shrimp begins to brown and peppers are al dente (tender-crisp).

7. Remove from heat, toss with tomatoes.

NUTRITION:

Calories: 529

Protein: 34g

Carbohydrates: 68g

Fats: 13g

73. Italian Shrimp and Broccoli

Preparation Time: 5 minutes

Cooking Time: 15 minutes

Servings: 1

INGREDIENTS:

2 cups raw chopped broccoli

(7 oz.) frozen and cooked shrimp (When cooked, each serving should yield one (7 oz)

½ cup (4 medium) cherry tomatoes, chopped

2 tablespoon of Lite Northern Italian with Basil & Romano

½ teaspoon freshly ground black pepper

1 tablespoon parmesan cheese; you may need it to be grated or shredded (optional condiment)

1 teaspoon olive oil

DIRECTIONS:

1. Thaw frozen shrimp. Just follow the directions on the package (about 5–7 minutes). In a skillet, heat olive oil and add broccoli and chopped cherry tomatoes; sauté until vegetables are al dente (tender-crisp).

2. Remove from heat, cover, and set aside. Spoon salad dressing into a skillet; add shrimp and black pepper. Sauté until shrimp are cooked (or opaque in color).

3. Combine shrimp and vegetables; cook an additional 2–3 minutes to reheat vegetables, if necessary. Place shrimp and vegetables on a plate, add parmesan cheese (optional condiment), and stir.

NUTRITION:

Calories: 529

Protein: 34g

Carbohydrates: 68g

Fats: 13g

74. Pan-"Fried" Catfish

Preparation Time: 5 minutes

Cooking Time: 10 minutes

Servings: 1

INGREDIENTS:

1–½ cups (½ large) summer squash, sliced

8 oz. wild catfish, raw; you may also opt for 6 oz. farmed catfish, raw (This should result in one 7-oz cooked wild catfish providing or one 5-oz cooked farmed catfish serving)

Non-stick cooking spray

1–½ cups (1 small-medium) zucchini, sliced

1/2 teaspoon olive oil

1/2 tablespoon low-fat mayonnaise, like Miracle Whip® or Kraft® light mayonnaise

1/3 teaspoon coriander leaves, chopped

1/2 teaspoon lime juice

1/16 teaspoon chili powder or ground chipotle chile pepper

DIRECTIONS:

1. Start with the tartar sauce by mixing mayonnaise, coriander, lime juice, and chili powder/chipotle pepper in a bowl.

2. Make sure to mix well; set aside for later use. Clean and chop zucchini and squash. Lightly brush catfish with olive oil.

3. Now, preheat a small non-stick skillet on medium-high heat. Later spray the skillet with a non-stick cooking spray can for 5–10 seconds.

4. Then, sauté the chopped vegetables until al dente (tender-crisp). Do not forget to remove vegetables from heat and cover-up to keep warm while cooking catfish. Place catfish (brushed with olive oil) in the pan, let it cook each side for 1 minute or until seared.

5. Next, lessen the heat to medium. Let it cook for 2–3 minutes on each side or until catfish flakes easily; use a fork. Lastly, serve cooked catfish with sautéed vegetables.

NUTRITION:

Calories: 151

Protein: 26g

Carbohydrates: 0g

Fats: 4.5g

75. Zesty Grilled Vegetables and Mahi-Mahi

Preparation Time: 5 minutes

Cooking Time: 15 minutes

Servings: 1

INGREDIENTS:

1 pound (16 oz.) raw mahi-mahi (should yield two (7 oz) cooked servings)

1 cup (1 small) zucchini with peel, sliced

1 cup (1 medium-large 3" x 2–¾") red bell pepper, sliced

1 cup (1 medium-large 3" x 2–¾") yellow bell pepper, sliced

¼ cup Newman's Own® Family Recipe Italian Dressing

1 serving of green

DIRECTIONS:

1. Preheat grill to medium heat. Place vegetables in a grill basket.

2. Grill 10 minutes or until al dente (tender-crisp), turning occasionally.

3. Then place fish on the grill and cook for 4–5 minutes on each side. You may also wait until fish flakes easily with a fork.

4. Next, place vegetables in a medium bowl. Also, add the dressing. You need to toss it for coating.

5. Divide the vegetables onto two plates and place one serving of mahi-mahi on each plate.

NUTRITION:

Calories: 340

Protein: 50g

Carbohydrates: 14g

Fats: 10g

Conclusion

The Optavia Diet can be effectively used for rapid weight loss compared to other plans simply because of the offer made by —lean and green‖ meals and its few calories. According to U.S. News and World Report, it listed Optavia on the number 2 position is the best diet for rapid weight loss. They tied with Keto, Atkins, and Weight Watchers. However, the 2019 U.S. News and World Report Best Diets positioned the Optavia Diet in number 31 in the list of Best Diets overall and graded it as 2.7 / 5.

Optavia doesn't require much-exerted energy compared to its competitors such as Weight Watchers (here, you will have to master a system of points) or keto (here, you must assess and closely track macronutrients).

The coaching component of Optavia can be compared to Jenny Craig and Weight Watchers, which urge users to register for meet-ups to get the necessary support.

Due to the highly processed nature of the majority of foods available on the Optavia diet, it could pose a threat or challenge compared to the variety of whole, fresh foods you can consume on more self-sustainable plans such as Atkins.

The Optavia diet enables weight loss through one-on-one coaching, low carb homemade meals, and low-calorie prepackaged diets.

Although the initial 5 & 1 Plan is quite limiting, the 3 & 3 maintenance phase enables fewer processed snacks and a wider variety of food, making it easier to lose weight and adhere to the program for sustenance in the long term.

Nevertheless, the diet is repetitive, costly, and doesn't cover all dietary needs. Another point is that extended calorie restriction may lead to nutrient deficiencies and other risky health concerns.

Although the program promotes fat loss and short-term weight loss, further research is required to evaluate the level of lifestyle changes it needs for long-term success.

CPSIA information can be obtained
at www.ICGtesting.com
Printed in the USA
LVHW011023140121
676458LV00012B/381

9 781801 454360